SO-BEZ-562

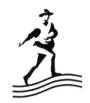

Chaiian Book Services s.a
Building #2
c W.M.S.C.

OTHER BOOKS BY KAPLAN MEDICAL

USMLE™ Step 1 Qbook

USMLE™ Step 2 CK Qbook

USMLE™ Step 3 Qbook

KAPLAN medical

USMLE™* Step 2 Clinical Skills

Simon & Schuster

NEW YORK · LONDON · SYDNEY · TORONTO

*USMLE™ is a joint program of the Federation of State Medical Boards of the United States, Inc. and the National Board of Medical Examiners.

Kaplan Publishing
Published by Simon & Schuster
1230 Avenue of the Americas
New York, New York 10020

Copyright © 2004 by Kaplan, Inc.

All rights reserved. No part of this book may be reproduced or transmitted in any form or by any means, electronic or mechanical, including photocopying, recording, or by any information storage and retrieval system, without the written permission of the Publisher, except where permitted by law.

For bulk sales to schools, colleges, and universities, please contact: Order Department, Simon and Schuster, 100 Front Street, Riverside, NJ 08075. Phone: (800) 223-2336. Fax: (800) 943-9831.

Kaplan® is a registered trademark of Kaplan, Inc.

The material in this book is up-to-date at the time of publication. However, the testmaker may have instituted changes in the test after this book was published. Be sure to carefully read the materials you receive when you register for the test.

If there are any important late-breaking developments—or any changes or corrections to the Kaplan test preparation materials in this book—we will post that information online at kaptest.com/publishing. Check to see if there is any information posted there regarding this book.

Kaplan Publishing
Executive Editor: Jennifer Farthing
Project Editor: Larissa Shmailo
Production Manager: Michael Shevlin
Cover Design: Cheung Tai

Manufactured in the United States of America
Published simultaneously in Canada

September 2004

10 9 8 7 6 5 4 3 2 1

ISBN: 0-7432-6240-9

AUTHOR

Elliott Wolfe, M.D., F.A.C.P.
Stanford University School of Medicine
Director, Office of Medical Student Professional Development
Adjunct Clinical Professor of Medicine

Content Editors

Rochelle Rothstein, M.D.
Senior Vice President
Kaplan Medical

Richard Friedland, D.P.M.
Executive Director of Curriculum
Kaplan Medical

Elissa Levy, M.D.

Marie Sicari, M.D.

Contributing Editors

Lisa Mellor, M.D.
Assistant Professor of Family Medicine
Robert Wood Johnson Medical School

Randi Bleier, R.N.
CS Manager
Kaplan Medical

Managing Editor

Kathlyn McGreevy

Production Manager

Michael Wolff

Contents

Preface

Congratulations on taking the first step toward passing your Step 2 Clinical Skills (CS) examination. Kaplan Medical has been preparing physicians for clinical skills exams since the introduction of the CSA in 1998. We have state-of-the-art clinical skills centers in Rutherford, NJ; Palo Alto, CA; and Chicago, IL.

The Step 2 CS primarily tests your proficiency in eliciting information from patients. Your basic clinical impression, as well as your initial thoughts on the diagnostic workup, comes into play. The Step 2 CS assesses these skills through the use of standardized patient encounters. During these encounters, you will usually have to perform a focused history and physical examination and write a patient note summarizing your findings. This book will teach you the methodology needed for success during these encounters.

Chapter 1 gives a broad, detailed overview about the USMLE Step 2 CS. It covers the entire examination process (score reporting, eligibility, registration, and fees, among others). The second chapter, titled "Doctor/Patient Relationships," focuses on a crucial component of the scoring: effective communication. Chapters 3, 4, and 5 walk you through taking the patient's medical history, performing the physical exam, and writing the patient note, respectively. Read through each of these chapters carefully, doing the clinical exercises (with suggested mnemonics for guidance) and checking against the answers found in Appendix V. They will help make all parts of the exam feel more natural to you. As you work through this book, note the areas that you are most weak in and practice until you feel more at ease. Further, we have helpful information in Section II: Appendices for you to reference when needed, such as common medical abbreviations, suggested phrasings of instructions for the physical exam, and much more.

Good luck on your exam.

Kaplan Medical

The USMLE™ Step 2 Clinical Skills Exam

Chapter One: **About the USMLE™ Step 2 Clinical Skills Exam**

ABOUT THE USMLE

The United States Medical Licensing Examination (USMLE) consists of three steps designed to assess a physician's ability to apply a broad spectrum of knowledge, concepts, and principles and to evaluate the physician's basic patient-centered skills.

- **Step 1 (multiple-choice exam)**—This exam is designed to test how well the examinee understands and applies concepts integral to the basic and clinical sciences.

- **Step 2 (two separate exams)**—The Step 2 Clinical Knowledge (CK) is a multiple-choice exam designed to determine whether the examinee possesses the medical knowledge and understanding of clinical science considered essential for the provision of patient care under supervision. The Step 2 Clinical Skills (CS) is a separate, "hands on" exam that tests the examinee's clinical and communication skills through his or her ability to gather information from standardized patients, perform a physical examination, communicate the findings to the patient, and write a student note.

- **Step 3 (multiple-choice exam)**—This exam assesses the examinee's ability to apply medical knowledge and the understanding of biomedical and clinical science essential for the unsupervised practice of medicine, with emphasis on patient management in ambulatory settings.

The results of the USMLE are reported to medical licensing authorities in the United States and its territories ("state boards") for use in granting the initial license to practice medicine. The examination serves to provide a common basis for evaluation of all candidates for licensure. The USMLE is sponsored by the Federation of State Medical Boards (FSMB) and the National Board of Medical Examiners (NBME).

OVERVIEW OF THE STEP 2 CS EXAM

Step 2 CS is a one-day live exam that resembles a physician's typical workday in a clinic, doctor's office, emergency department, and/or hospital setting in the United States. You have 15 minutes to examine each "standardized patient" (SP), who is an actor chosen from a broad range of age and racial and ethnic backgrounds and trained to portray a real patient. You are expected to communicate with the SPs in a professional and empathetic manner (in short, to establish a rapport with them) while simultaneously eliciting important historic information and performing a physical examination. You must answer questions from the SPs, tell them what diagnoses are being considered, provide counseling when appropriate, and inform them what tests will be ordered to clarify their diagnoses. After each encounter, you must record pertinent history and physical examination findings, list diagnostic impressions, and outline plans for further evaluation, if necessary.

The purpose of USMLE Step 2 CS is to test your clinical and communication skills. The medical community believes this to be a skill set necessary for better patient safety, compliance, and satisfaction. Therefore, the cases covered by this test will cover common and important situations that a physician is likely to encounter in a general ambulatory clinic in the United States.

DESCRIPTION OF THE STEP 2 CS EXAM

Each Step 2 Clinical Skills Evaluation Center simulates a large medical clinic. There are 24 fully equipped examination rooms. On each examination room door, you will find an instruction sheet containing basic information about the case, including the patient's age, chief complaint, and vital signs. The instruction sheet will also list the tasks that you are expected to perform.

After reading the instruction sheet and taking notes, you should knock on the door and begin your encounter with the standardized patient (SP), just as you would with a real patient. In the course of the examination, you will go through 11 or 12 different exam rooms and will encounter a different case in each room. Eleven of these encounters will be scored. The unscored patient encounter is included for piloting new cases and other research purposes. However, you should treat every single encounter on test day as a scored encounter.

The Patient Encounter

You will have **15 minutes** for each patient encounter and will meet 11 or 12 SPs. During each encounter, you must:

- Establish rapport with the standardized patient.
- Obtain a pertinent patient history.
- Perform a focused physical examination.
- Demonstrate a satisfactory level of communication and interpersonal skills, as well as spoken English language skills.
- Document findings and diagnostic impressions.

As noted above, on the door to each of the examination rooms is posted some basic information (e.g., patient's name, age, presenting complaint, pertinent vital signs) for you to review before walking in. You may assume all the information is accurate, but if clinically indicated, you may repeat some of the vital signs, such as pulse and blood pressure.

Because the examination is standardized, all examinees receive the same information when they ask standardized patients the same or similar questions.

Note that certain parts of the physical examination must not be done on the exam. These include rectal, pelvic, genitourinary, female breast, or corneal reflex examinations. If you believe such exams are indicated, you should include them in the proposed diagnostic workup. Eventually, however, synthetic models, mannequins, or simulators may be offered as alternative formats for assessment of some of these sensitive examination areas.

The Patient Note

After each encounter, record a patient note, including:

- Relevant history.
- Physical examination findings.
- Diagnostic impressions.
- Plans for further evaluation, if necessary.

You will have **10 minutes** to write your note.

Step 2 CS Strategy

You won't know which of the patients you see will count toward your score. Treat every patient as if the encounter will be scored.

Step 2 CS Strategy

It is impossible to conduct a full physical examination and obtain a lengthy patient history in 15 minutes. The key words for this time-critical exam are "pertinent" and "focused."

Note

There's a second copy of the instruction sheet in the examination room to which you can refer.

Step 2 CS at a Glance

Total Examination Length: 8 hours with two breaks (30 minutes; 15 minutes)

Patient Encounters: 11 or 12 (11 are scored)

Length of Each Patient Encounter: 15 minutes

Time Allotted for Writing Each Patient Note: 10 minutes

WHAT IS TESTED ON THE STEP 2 CS

Most cases are specially designed to test the type of history-taking and focused examination that demonstrate your ability to list and pursue possible diagnoses. Some cases, however, may focus only on history taking or on physical examination. All of the SPs will be adults, although some of the scenarios may involve a parent of a child or a sibling of an elderly patient. In these cases, physical examination of the patient will not be required. However, you will still have relevant information and instructions and will be expected to take a history, ask questions, and write a patient note.

The clinical skills examination measures skills that cannot be measured by traditional multiple-choice exams. Step 2 CS assesses whether you can demonstrate—on the spot—the fundamental clinical skills essential to safe and effective patient care under supervision. These clinical skills include taking a relevant medical history, performing an appropriate and focused physical examination, communicating effectively with the patient, clearly and accurately documenting the findings and diagnostic hypotheses from the clinical encounter, and ordering appropriate initial diagnostic studies.

Presentation categories include but are not limited to:

- Cardiovascular
- Constitutional
- Gastrointestinal
- Genitourinary
- Musculoskeletal
- Neurologic
- Psychiatric
- Respiratory
- Women's Health

Note

Even though this is a simulated exam, be sure to perform physical examination maneuvers correctly and expect that there may be positive physical findings in some encounters. Accept any positive findings as real and factor them into your evolving physical diagnoses.

Note

Based on the patient's presenting complaint, doorway information, and additional information you obtain during the history, be sure to consider all possible diagnoses, then explore the relevant ones as time permits.

HOW THE STEP 2 CS IS SCORED

The Patient Encounter

The SPs you encounter during the exam are trained to document your actions in a fair and consistent manner. Immediately following each patient encounter, the standardized patient fills out checklists that document the inquiries you made and maneuvers you performed during the encounter.

The **history-taking checklist** includes the inquiries you are expected to make in the course of taking the patient's history for a particular case. The **physical examination checklist** includes the maneuvers you should perform during the course of a physical examination for the particular case. Your technique in doing these maneuvers is also observed by the SP. Additionally, carefully developed **rating scales** are used by the SPs, who are highly trained in their use, to assess **communication**, **interpersonal skills**, and **English speaking skills**.

The Patient Note

Your ability to document your findings from the patient encounter, your diagnostic impressions, and the initial patient workup will be evaluated by physician raters. You will be rated on the quality of documentation of important positive and negative findings from the history and physical examination, as well as your listed differential diagnoses and diagnostic assessment plans.

SCORE REPORTING

Performance on Step 2 CS is reported as *pass* or *fail*. Examinees who fail receive performance profiles covering the strengths and weaknesses of their performance across the components of Step 2 CS.

The checklists and rating methods for the patient encounter and patient note result in three primary components that are assessed for the Step 2 CS:

1. The Integrated Clinical Encounter (ICE), which includes history-taking and physical examination, as well as completion of the patient note
2. Communication/Interpersonal Skills (CIS)
3. Spoken English Proficiency (SEP)

You must pass all three in a single administration to receive a *pass* score on the Step 2 CS.

ELIGIBILITY

To be eligible to take the Step 2 CS, you must be in one of the following categories at the time of application and on test day:

- A medical student officially enrolled in, or a graduate of, a U.S. or Canadian medical school program leading to the M.D. degree that is accredited by the Liaison Committee on Medical Education (LCME)
- A medical student officially enrolled in, or a graduate of, a U.S. medical school program leading to the D.O. degree that is accredited by the American Osteopathic Association (AOA)
- A medical student officially enrolled in, or a graduate of, a medical school outside the United States and Canada and eligible for examination by the ECFMG for its certificate

---

Step 2 CS Strategy

There will be more than one diagnosis for most Step 2 CS cases.

USMLE EXAM SEQUENCING

Students and graduates of LCME- and AOA-accredited medical schools may take Step 1, Step 2 CK, and Step 2 CS in any sequence.

Students and graduates of medical schools outside the United States and Canada must pass Step 1 before registering for Step 2 CS.

REGISTRATION AND SCHEDULING FOR THE STEP 2 CS EXAM

Students and graduates of medical schools **in the United States and Canada** accredited by the Liaison Committee on Medical Education or the American Osteopathic Association may register for the Step 2 CS through:

> **NBME**
> Examinee Support Services
> 3750 Market Street
> Philadelphia, PA 19104-3190
>
> Website: http://www.nbme.org
> Telephone: (215) 590-9700
> Fax: (215) 590-9457
> E-mail: webmail@nbme.org

You may use one application to apply for Step 1 and both components of Step 2 at the same time.

Students and graduates of medical schools **outside the United States and Canada** may register for the Step 2 CS through:

> **ECFMG**
> 3624 Market Street
> Philadelphia, PA 19104-2685
>
> Website: http://www.ecfmg.org
> Telephone: (215) 386-5900
> Fax: (215) 386-9196
> E-mail: info@ecfmg.org

International students may also complete a paper application (Form 106S). You can download Form 106S from the ECFMG website or request a photocopy from ECFMG.

Eligibility Periods

Applicants registered for Step 2 CS are assigned a 12-month eligibility period that begins on the date that their registration information is entered into the Step 2 CS scheduling system. The eligibility period is listed on the Step 2 CS Scheduling Permit. You must take the exam during your eligibility period. If you do not take the exam within your eligibility period, you must reapply, including payment of the examination fee.

Scheduling Your Test Date

Once you have received your Scheduling Permit, you can access Step 2 CS scheduling through the website of your registration entity (ECFMG or NBME). To schedule an appointment, you must select a test date and a test center. The date must fall within your eligibility period. There are AM and PM sessions. Testing appointments are available on a first-come, first-served basis.

Note

For students and graduates of international medical schools, Step 2 CS will replace the ECFMG Clinical Skills Assessment (CSA®) for purposes of ECFMG certification.

Note

Although there are no deadlines for taking the Step 2 CS, don't forget to check the National Resident Matching Program (NRMP) and Graduate Medical Education (GME) programs for their deadlines.

After you confirm your testing appointment, you will be able to print a confirmation notice from the scheduling system. The confirmation notice includes your scheduled test date, session (AM or PM), test center, and other important information.

If you are unable to schedule online, call (215) 966-3574 (9:00 AM to 5:00 PM Eastern Time in the United States, Monday through Friday) to speak to a representative who will access the online scheduling system for you.

Rescheduling

If you are unable to take the exam on your scheduled test date or at your scheduled test center, you can cancel your scheduled testing appointment and reschedule for a different available date and/or center *within your eligibility period*. There is no limit on the number of times you can cancel and reschedule your testing appointment. However, a rescheduling fee is charged for each rescheduled test (see below). If you cancel and do not reschedule within your eligibility period, you must reapply, including repayment of the examination fee, to take the exam.

FEES

Exam fee

- $975 USD for U.S. and Canadian medical school students and graduates
- $1,200 USD for international medical school students and graduates

Cancellation/Rescheduling fees

- $50 rescheduling fee if canceled 30 days or more before (but not including) the scheduled test date
- $150 rescheduling fee if canceled during the 30-day period before (but not including) the scheduled test date
- $400 rescheduling fee if the test appointment is not canceled.

Fees are subject to change. For updates, refer to the USMLE website.

STEP 2 CS EVALUATION CENTERS

Step 2 CS will be administered at regional Clinical Skills Evaluation Centers (CSEC) at the following locations:

Clinical Skills Evaluation Center–Atlanta
Two Crown Center
1745 Phoenix Boulevard, Suite 500
Atlanta, GA 30349

Clinical Skills Evaluation Center–Chicago
Crossroads Center at O'Hare
6th Floor
8501 West Higgins Road
Chicago, IL 60018

Clinical Skills Evaluation Center–Houston
400 North Belt
400 North Sam Houston Parkway
Suite 700
Houston, TX 77060

Clinical Skills Evaluation Center–Los Angeles
Pacific Corporate Towers
13th Floor
100 N. Sepulveda Boulevard
El Segundo, CA 90245

Clinical Skills Evaluation Center–Philadelphia
3624 Market Street
Philadelphia, PA 19104

ON EXAMINATION DAY

The Step 2 CS exam begins with an onsite orientation session in which you have the opportunity to ask questions and use the diagnostic equipment available in the examination rooms. You'll also be informed of test rules and procedures. *Be sure not to miss this session.* In addition, note carefully the following advice and information:

- Arrive at the test center 30 minutes before the scheduled examination.
- Bring your Scheduling Permit and a government-issued form of identification (e.g., driver's license or passport).
- You will be given a small storage cubicle in which you may place personal belongings. These cubicles are not secure, so do not bring valuables.
- Wear comfortable, professional clothing *and a white laboratory coat.*
- Bring your own stethoscope; all other equipment is provided at the center.
- Do not bring electronic paging devices, personal digital assistants, cellular telephones, or any other communication or photographic devices. Take this rule seriously: Breaking it is considered misconduct and may jeopardize your test.
- Follow the instructions of staff members (wearing name tags) at all times.
- Once the orientation has started, you may not leave that area until the examination is over.

- The examination lasts about 8 hours. There are two breaks: one 30-minute break and one 15-minute break. A light meal is also provided. You may bring your own food, provided that no refrigeration or preparation is required. There are vending machines for drinks. During breaks, you are free to relax and use the restrooms.

- You may not discuss the cases with your fellow examinees at any time.

- Conversation among examinees and with patients in any language other than English is prohibited at all times.

- Proctors will monitor all examinee activity.

- On the day of the Step 2 CS examination, you may be asked to sign documents intended to confirm your understanding and willingness to abide by USMLE policies and procedures. You may also be asked to complete demographic and feedback surveys after the examination.

RETAKING AN EXAMINATION

If you fail or don't complete Step 2 CS, you may retake it, but you must reapply and pay all test fees again. You may not retake Step 2 CS within 60 days of your last attempt. Additionally, you cannot take Step 2 CS more than three times in any 12-month period. Previous ECFMG CSA attempts will be counted as attempts on Step 2 CS. See the USMLE website for policies regarding the retaking of USMLE Steps.

EXAMINEES WITH DISABILITIES

Reasonable accommodations will be made for USMLE examinees with disabilities who are covered under the Americans with Disabilities Act (ADA). If you wish to apply for test accommodations, you must send your official request and documentation at the same time that you apply for the exam. See the USMLE website for more information.

FOR STUDENTS AND GRADUATES OF INTERNATIONAL MEDICAL SCHOOLS

For students and graduates of international medical schools, Step 2 CS replaces the ECFMG Clinical Skills Assessment (CSA®) for purposes of ECFMG Certification. This has resulted in changes to some policies and procedures related to ECFMG Certification, including the required exams, the time limits for completing these exams, and ECFMG's revalidation and permanent validation policies. Other changes may also take place. If you are seeking ECFMG Certification, you should:

- Review the Step 2 CS information on the USMLE website.

- Monitor the ECFMG website and the USMLE website. New information regarding Step 2 CS policies and procedures will be published as it becomes available.

- Subscribe to *The ECFMG Reporter*, ECFMG's free e-mail newsletter. ECFMG publishes updates on the transition to Step 2 CS in *The ECFMG Reporter* as new information becomes available.

- Review the information on the transition to Step 2 CS in the ECFMG *Information Booklet* and the USMLE *Bulletin of Information*, available at the ECFMG and USMLE websites.

FOR MORE INFORMATION

- See the USMLE *Bulletin of Information* and the USMLE website at USMLE.org. Changes can occur after the *Bulletin* is released, so monitor the USMLE website for the most current information about the test.

- Refer to the website of your registration entity (Educational Commission for Foreign Medical Graduates [ECFMG®] for students and graduates of international medical schools; the National Board of Medical Examiners [NBME®] for students and graduates of U.S. and Canadian medical schools).

- View the orientation video, available on the USMLE website.

- Review the Step 2 CS CD you will receive when you register.

Chapter Two: **Doctor/Patient Relationships**

THE COMMUNICATION/INTERPERSONAL SKILLS (CIS) COMPONENT OF THE STEP 2 CS EXAM

Effective communication skills provide the link between the various parts of the exam by allowing you to efficiently obtain the information needed during the brief encounter time. On the basis of the cooperative responses of the patient, you can determine which body systems to focus on during the physical exam. The patient will become less anxious and more compliant with your requests when you give clear instructions, explain what you are doing each step of the way, and assure the patient that each maneuver is medically important. Likewise, in closing the encounter, summarize your findings from the history, confirming their accuracy with the patient. Pertinent findings from the physical exam might be mentioned in the summary as well. Answering any questions the patient may have also gives you a final opportunity to reinforce your competency. Finally, armed with adequate positive and negative findings from the history and physical, you will be able to produce the patient note more quickly, with better organization, and with greater accuracy.

The communication skills, along with the history and physical exam, are scored by the SP, who checks off items on a computerized list as soon as you leave the room. In addition, the SP rates the comprehensibility of your spoken English in terms of pronunciation, grammar, and degree of ease in understanding what you said. SPs are thoroughly trained to reduce any existing bias toward accent and country of origin. But remember to speak clearly and carefully and to rephrase what you have said if the patient seems not to have understood. The CIS score is an average of the eleven *scored* encounters. Because of this method of scoring, you could perform awkwardly or ineffectively in one or two encounters, yet still succeed on the whole exam if you communicate more effectively in other encounters.

Using the interpersonal skills checklist, the SP rates your skills in *interviewing and collecting information, counseling and delivering information, establishing rapport,* and *maintaining a positive personal manner.* Each of the skill areas involves a handful of key characteristics that are important for effective communication in general. Mastery in each area can be achieved by plenty of practice with actual patients or with those who are role-playing a medical case. To deepen and expand self-awareness, seek feedback from the role-playing patient regarding his or her perception of your interpersonal skills.

TIMING THE PATIENT ENCOUNTER

Time management on the Step 2 CS is crucial. In Table 2-1, we have listed the suggested time you should spend in each stage of the encounter. We recommend that you spend 1 minute outside the room reviewing the doorway information. The next 7 minutes should be spent greeting the patient, eliciting the chief complaint, supporting history of the present illness, and related review of systems. Following your hand-washing (15 to 30 seconds), you should spend 5 minutes performing a focused physical exam. Finally, you will need 2 minutes to explain to the patient your findings and answer any questions he or she may have.

Note

For each encounter on the exam, you will get a 5-minute warning. You should be in the middle of performing the physical exam when you get this announcement.

Kaplan Medical Strategy

To help you monitor time during the encounters, turn your watch to the inside of your wrist so that you can glance at it without the patient noticing.

Table 2-1. Timing the Patient Encounter

Task	Minutes
Introductory (doorway) information	1
CC and HPI	7
Physical examination	5
Closing	2

CONDUCTING THE INTERVIEW

Entering the Room

Before knocking on the door and entering the room, concentrate on how you will greet the patient using the usual social amenities. Knock on the door, wait an instant, and then open the door just enough to ask the patient's permission to enter. It is proper to introduce yourself using title, first, and last name; for example: "Hello, Ms. Cleary, I'm Dr. Ron Singh, a senior medical student." Never refer to any patient by their first name only. Remain consistently aware of words you are using during this and all phases of the interview; it is often disquieting to patients if physicians use too informal or personal statements, e.g., "How are you?" or "I am pleased to meet you." Patients are visiting the medical office or hospital because of an important concern and may be fearful of the visit; therefore, more lighthearted phrases are best avoided. A patient may be placed at ease by asking "How can I help you today?" or referring to the symptom noted on the doorway: "I understand you have a severe headache—tell me about it." Patients know you have taken an interest in their concerns when you refer to information they have provided, and this enables rapport to be rapidly established.

If a patient offers to shake your hand, returning the gesture is often appropriate. For cultural reasons, it is better to not offer the handshake because not all patients are comfortable with this form of greeting. Of course, physicians and patients are also aware that handshaking may transmit infections.

When you enter the room during the CS examination, a draping sheet will be folded and available on an adjacent chair or the examining table. Before you sit down and start the medical interview, apply the drape to cover the patient's lower limbs.

Interviewing and Collecting Information

For *interviewing and collecting information*, a highly valued characteristic is the ability to ask *clearly worded questions*. In general, the more words in the question, the harder it is to follow, especially if you speak English with an accent that is different from the patient's. Use as *few words* as needed to express an idea, and use *short, nonmedical words*. Any person with any level of education or sophistication should be able to easily understand what you are asking and should therefore be able to answer easily. Likewise, speaking relatively slowly improves the chances of being understood in any language, with any accent. If medical terminology must be used, explain the term immediately in *lay language* before the patient has to ask what the term means. If you wait for the patient to ask for an explanation, you may very well not be given credit by the SP for having maintained lay language. An appropriate use of medical language would be naming a particular disease with an explanation of it in simple terms. For example, "I think you may have an infection of the gallbladder. The medical name for this condition is cholecystitis." Similarly, when suggesting which tests you would like to have administered, say, "I'd like you to have a blood test," rather than "I'd like to run a CBC with differential." To the opposite extreme, do not use slang. Slang gives the impression that the physician is less than professional. Leave it up to the patients to use slang terms. If they do, and you don't know what the term means, simply ask, "What do you mean by that?" Asking for clarification is a sound method in communication skills.

Clarification and other questioning techniques

Clarification is also a way of *verifying* with the patient that you have heard a response correctly. It is wise to *paraphrase* throughout the interviewing process. Shortly after eliciting the chief complaint (by having asked, "What caused you to come in today?") and obtaining answers to a few other followup questions, it is a good idea to quickly reflect the main points to the patient. Afterward, ask, "Is that correct?" If you've misunderstood any part of the response, the patient can then clarify. Paraphrasing of this sort will assist you greatly in your clinical reasoning.

Paraphrase

Here are some examples of reflection and paraphrasing:

Doctor: "I see you're wearing an Ace bandage on your wrist. What happened?"

Patient: "Oh, I hurt my wrist playing tennis yesterday."

Doctor: (Nodding) "Playing tennis."

Doctor: "I see you're wearing an Ace bandage on your wrist. What happened there?"

Patient: "Oh, I hurt my wrist playing pool yesterday."

Doctor: (Nodding) "Playing polo."

Patient: "No, no—playing pool."

Doctor: "Oh, okay. Playing pool."

Doctor: "Have you had any change in your weight lately?"

Patient: "Yeah, I've lost about seven or eight pounds."

Doctor: "Over what period of time?"

Patient: "Let's see—over about the past two months."

Doctor: "So for the past couple of months, you've lost about seven or eight pounds."

Patient: "Uh-huh."

Doctor: "Has your weight changed any lately?"

Patient: "Yes, I must've lost about seven or eight pounds."

Doctor: "Over what length of time?"

Patient: "About two months."

Doctor: "So you've lost about seven or eight pounds over the past two weeks?"

Patient: "No, not two weeks; it's been about two months."

Doctor: "Oh, two months. All right."

In addition to using simple, short sentences, along with paraphrase and occasional verification, you may need to refine your questioning techniques. One important technique is phrasing the question in the *affirmative mode* rather than the negative. Ask, "Do you smoke?" rather than, "You don't smoke, do you?" Questions phrased in the affirmative convey a nonjudgmental tone, encouraging the patient to answer more candidly, without fear of being blamed for medically significant behaviors like smoking, using recreational drugs, drinking alcohol, or having multiple sexual partners. The physician needs to get the facts, and so must ask questions in such a way that the patient feels at ease in confiding what can sometimes be embarrassing admissions.

Not only should the followup questions be cast in a *neutral tone*, they should also be phrased in a *specific* way to elicit specific responses. If you ask, "Do you have any other symptoms?," the SP will probably say, "Like what?" On the other hand, you should already have in mind some associated symptoms, if you ask, "Do you have diarrhea?" or "Have you been feeling nauseated?" or "Was there any blood in your vomit?" the patient can more readily answer questions without trying to guess what you had in mind. These kinds of questions, which are called *close-ended*, should comprise the bulk of queries during the history.

Unlike *close-ended questions,* which generally call for a one- or two-word answer, *open-ended questions* call for a longer, more detailed response, usually a sentence or two in which the patient describes or narrates something in his or her own words. A typical open-ended question would be, "How would you describe your pain?" or "Can you explain that further?" or "What happened right before that?" These questions are usually posed at the beginning of a line of interrogatives and are then followed by the more specific, often quantitative, direct questions. A fine balance can be struck between these two modes of questioning so that the patient gets to express what is important to him or her personally, while allowing you to obtain accurate data in a timely fashion.

It is of utmost importance to ask only *one question at a time*, then wait for the patient to answer. Don't barrage the patient with a string of questions: "Has anyone in your family ever had high blood pressure, high cholesterol, strokes, or any heart condition that you know of?" Separate these items and ask them one at a time. Otherwise, the patient becomes confused and feels rushed. In addition, you will have used poor time management in running questions together in this way, for the SP will probably say, "What? Which one? I'm confused." Then the candidate must start all over again, this time waiting for the patient to respond point by point. Worse yet, the SP may respond only to the final question in the string of questions, thus misleading you into thinking that the answer applies to all the previous parts as well, and so undermining your clinical reasoning.

Don't interrupt

Similarly, *do not interrupt* a patient's answer unless absolutely necessary. Let the patient finish his or her answer, even if there are pauses and silences while the patient thinks or processes feelings. Wait. Grant the patient the proper respect of being heard fully. If the question has hit on a sensitive issue and the patient becomes teary, stand there in silence; better yet, sit down and quietly wait for the patient to regain composure. Gently gaze at the patient with a compassionate expression in your eyes. It is permissible to convey supportiveness by resting your hand for one second gently on the patient's shoulder or upper arm (not the leg or hand, and do not pat). *Silence* is one of the least invasive interviewing techniques, one that encourages the patient to open up and share more freely. Wait for three full seconds before expressing *empathy* in some verbal way, such as saying slowly and quietly, while making eye contact: "This must have been a very difficult time for you." Pause in silence for two more seconds, then add, "Ms. Smith, would you be willing to share with me what happened at that time?" If the patient senses your genuine concern, he or she is much more likely to open up. Don't worry about the lack of time in a sensitive case like grieving or depression; never lose sight of the human connection. The Step 2 CS is primarily a test of your interpersonal communication skills. And remember that the Step 2

CS cases are carefully planned to take approximately 15 minutes, including any expressions of emotion, or hesitation, on the part of the standardized patient.

Of course, it may sometimes be necessary to interrupt the patient. For example, the patient may be talking on and on about irrelevant matters, such as her boyfriend's friend's sister who is on drugs. In such a case, the physician may gain the patient's trust even more strongly by firmly interrupting to *refocus* on the patient. Cut in whenever the patient hesitates slightly, look the patient straight in the eyes and say, "Excuse me for interrupting, Ms. Jones." Next, *acknowledge* whatever the patient was talking about by stating, "I know these things have really been troubling you." Then bring the focus back to the patient: "However, right now I want to focus completely on *you*." Chances are Ms. Jones will feel honored and pleased that someone cares enough to want to focus on her.

Transition

Transitions are like signposts, alerting the patient that you are ready to move into a new area of questioning during the history; they also let the patient know that you are moving from the history to the physical, and then to the closing. Transitional statements allow the patient to follow along with the logic of your inquiry and thus help keep the communication clear. By conveying an impression of orderly thinking, transitions foster the patient's confidence and trust in the doctor's judgment. Additionally, transitional sentences encourage the patient to be more cooperative as well as to answer questions more readily.

Appropriate places to give a transitional statement are before the *past medical history*; before the *sexual and social histories*; before the *family history*; before the *physical exam*; during the physical exam as you proceed from *maneuver to maneuver*; and before the *closing*. The following are some examples:

Before the past medical history:

"Okay, Mr. Green, now I'm going to ask you some questions about your health in general."

Before the sexual history:

"All right, now I need to ask you some personal questions so that I may understand your health in general. Whatever you tell me will be kept confidential."

Before the social history:

"Thank you. Now let me ask you about your work, family, and social life."

Before asking questions about smoking, alcohol, and recreational drug use:

"Okay, now I need to get some information about your lifestyle."

Before the family history:

"Now let's talk about your family's health."

Before the physical exam:

"All right, thanks for answering all these questions. Now I'll need to examine you, so I'll just wash my hands. Excuse me. Okay, Mr. Green, let's begin by _____."

During the physical exam:

"Now I need to look in your throat to see if there's any redness or swelling."

Before the closing:

"Okay then, now I'd like to sit down and talk over what I think so far. First let me summarize…"

Summary

Summary is similar to paraphrasing, but it reflects more items of information to the patient. It is wise to summarize the most significant data gathered during the history once you have completed the physical exam.

Just before you share your diagnostic impression with the patient, say something like the following:

> Doctor: "All right, Ms. Cooper. Now I'd like to talk over what I'm considering so far. First let me summarize. You told me that you have had _____ over the past month; you've also _____. You said that _____ and that _____. Your sister and mother have both been treated for _____. In the physical exam, I observed that _____ and _____."

After this short summary, you are now ready to share your diagnostic impression with the patient in words such as these:

> "So, Ms. Cooper, I think that this problem may involve your _____. It's most likely _____."

Finish with tests suggested and possible questions on the part of the patient.

Closing and Delivering Information

Your skill level is determined by both the statements used to end the interview and other informative statements made earlier during both the history and physical exam. The *organization* of your interview in fairly distinct sections of history of present illness, past medical history, sexual history, OB/GYN, social history, and family history has established the pattern for an equally *orderly and satisfying closing*. Now you may summarize the most significant features of the history and physical, share your preliminary diagnostic impression, let the patient know what you would like to have him or her do next—such as take certain diagnostic tests (e.g., blood, urine, x-rays)—and find out if the patient has any questions to ask you.

Expect to be asked at least one rather challenging question. Especially if you mention something that has alarmed the patient, he or she is likely to ask, "Does this mean I'll have to be hospitalized?" or "Will this require surgery?" or "Are you telling me I may die soon?" Always respond to these expressions of vulnerability and fear in an *appropriately reassuring way*, not with premature or false statements. It would be a false reassurance to say, "Oh no, don't worry, you'll be fine!" Worse yet, "Oh no, this isn't important. You'll get over it." These statements are not only possibly false, they also minimize the suffering and anxiety of the patient to whom every aspect of the experience is disturbing.

Instead, assure the patient that you will be very careful and thorough in determining what he or she has and that you will definitely help him or her through this difficult experience. "As soon as we know precisely what you have, we'll sit down together and go over the various treatment options. So, first, let's get the tests started, and then we'll go from there." In a psychiatric case, such as depression or anxiety disorder, you may also suggest the possibility of peer support groups, counseling, or minor changes in daily habits. You would not write these down on the patient note, but it shows kindly and sincere concern to make such suggestions in the context of the encounter itself.

The SP may be cooperative and easy or grumpy and difficult. Never deny the patient's beliefs, no matter how unreasonable they may seem to you. (The Step 2 CS is designed to test your interpersonal and communication skills through a variety of interesting medical cases and patient personalities. The more you relish the opportunity to communicate clearly under all circumstances with kindness and human decency, the greater your success on this challenging exam.)

Rapport and Nonverbal Communication

Perhaps the most important factor in increasing the patient's compliance in actual clinical practice is a positive doctor-patient relationship. This phrase refers to the quality of *rapport* or *connectedness* between the physician and patient. A sense of genuine *concern and caring* is conveyed by a variety of sometimes subtle signals, both verbal and physical. In the United States, for instance, crossing of the arms in front of one's chest is a sign of closing out the other person, perhaps even a sign of resistance or distrust in the presence of another. If you catch yourself holding your clipboard as a shield across your chest with crossed arms, gently drop your hands down, and hold the clipboard loosely at your side. If you catch yourself talking too rapidly and loudly, slow down your pacing and lower your volume a bit; otherwise, you may unknowingly push the patient away with these subtle signs of aggression. Stand so that your patient can see you without straining, usually at a 45-degree angle, slightly off to the side. The patient should not have to turn his or her head to try to see you. Never stand behind the patient during the history or the closing. Look the patient comfortably in the eyes. Shifting your eyes around the room, avoiding looking directly at the patient, may communicate a lack of self-confidence. Standing too close or too far away may suggest either a stance of aggression or timidity, respectively. As a general rule, 2 feet is about right for personal proximity in the American culture.

An attitude of *composure, calm, and clarity* is wonderful in the patient encounter. The blending of lively interest in the medical aspects of the case with a sincere liking for the human person right in front of you is remarkably soothing for the worried patient. Your confident, nonconceited manner helps inspire the patient's confidence in you. The best way to stay calm under pressure is to *focus attention solely on the patient*, not on yourself as a performer. Watch the patient carefully. Be a good observer. Notice every detail. Ask questions. Listen. In the Step 2 CS, take every slight bit of evidence as a clue. A bandaged wrist may suggest domestic violence; a bruise on the upper arm of an elderly patient may indicate elder abuse. If the patient coughs into a handkerchief, ask to see it; there may be blood on it. Remember, the SP will not volunteer the very piece of information that could guide your clinical reasoning in a new direction. You will need to be a careful observer and ask questions accordingly.

Your *attention to detail* and your *verbal acknowledgment* of significant information solidify the bridge of genuine concern between you and the patient. *Support the patient* physically by extending the leg rest or by helping him or her to turn over. Acknowledge the pain he or she may be feeling: "You seem to be experiencing a lot of pain right now. Is there anything I can do to help you feel more comfortable?" Keep your eyes on your patient. Observe the patient's face for signs of discomfort or change of mood and comment on these changes. The SPs are well trained to portray feelings through facial expression. Nothing is an accident in the Step 2 CS. The rapport you establish through these simple expressions of empathy and support will earn you the positive regard of the patient.

Step 2 CS Strategy

High-rapport physicians:

1. Wash their hands in front of the patient

2. Sit down facing the patient

3. Are aware of their facial expression

4. Lean toward the patient

5. Nod their head periodically

6. Keep upper limbs unfolded and comfortable

7. Consult the medical record

8. Vary patterns of gaze without staring

9. Move from time to time, rather than sit stiffly

EVALUATION OF PERSONAL MANNER

The standardized patients will evaluate interpersonal and communication skills through the use of a checklist. Table 2-2 is designed to give you an idea of what could be included on a communication/interpersonal skills checklist. The following pages present a detailed description of each item.

Kaplan Medical's Five Essentials

1) Introduction—sets the tone for the encounter

2) Empathy—reflects the patient's feelings

3) Reassurance—aids the patient's feelings

4) Paraphrasing—clarifies patient's information and allows note taking while paying attention to the patient

5) Closing—crucial for exam success

Table 2-2. Communication Skills Checklist

No	Yes	Interpersonal/Communication Skills Feature
		1. Examinee **knocked** before entering
		2. Appeared professional in **dress/grooming/hygiene**
		3. **Introduced self** by name
		4. Made comfortable **eye contact**
		5. Focused **attention and concentration** on patient
		6. Conveyed a **respectful and nonjudgmental** attitude
		7. Used appropriate **draping** technique
		8. Used **transitional** phrases and references
		9. Expressed **empathy** (reflected patient's feelings) and made appropriate **reassurances**
		10. Gave patient time to think and answer **without interrupting**
		11. Asked **open-ended** questions
		12. Used **nonleading** questions
		13. Asked **one question at a time** (clear and concise)
		14. Used **lay language** (volunteered explanation)
		15. Effectively **listened** and **paraphrased** information throughout the encounter
		16. Was **connected** and **purposeful** during the physical examination
		17. **Summarized** significant information in closing, and clearly explained **diagnostic plans**
		18. Placed patient **at ease** and communicated information **without alarming** the patient
		19. **Asked** if patient had questions, and **answered promptly**

Interpersonal Skills Checklist: Explanation of Each Item

1. Examinee knocked before entering

Knock before coming into the examining room. By knocking first, you alert the patient that someone is about to intrude on his or her privacy. Knocking is thus a first step in building *trust* and showing *respect*. Wait until patient says "come in" before entering.

2. Appeared professional in dress/grooming/hygiene

- Make sure your white coat is clean and neat.
- Wear comfortable, conservative clothing. It is suggested that men wear trousers, a dress shirt, a tie, and dark shoes; and that women wear slacks or a skirt, low-heeled and closed-toe shoes, and conservative jewelry.
- Pull hair back away from face, trim nails, and use no products with scents (such as hairspray, perfume, or cologne).
- Make sure there are no body odors or stale odors in your clothing.

3. Introduced self by name

- You are given credit for introducing yourself by name and for identifying your role in the hospital. For example, "Let me introduce myself. My name is Dr. Smith. I'm a doctor here in the hospital."
- Address all male patients as Mr. Jones, for example, and all female patients as Ms. Jones, for example—regardless of age or marital status. By making a cordial introduction, you set a tone of *friendliness* and *positive rapport*.

4. Made comfortable eye contact

- Look directly and easily into the patient's eyes throughout most of the encounter. Of course, at times, you will be required to look elsewhere, such as at the clipboard notes or into the patient's ears. However, even during the physical exam, while palpating the abdomen, for example, observe the patient's face for any signs of pain or discomfort. In general, if you seem embarrassed to make eye contact and avoid doing so, or if you look distractedly around the room, you will not be given credit. Comfortable eye contact demonstrates your self-confidence in the presence of strangers and thus reinforces a sense of trust and credibility.
- *Position* yourself so that the patient can see you. For example, if the patient is lying down facing the wall, move around to that side to face the patient. You may want to sit down at certain points to be more *aligned* with the patient for better eye contact.

5. Focused attention and concentration on patient

- If you look repeatedly at your watch, credit may not be given. Turn your watch inside the wrist so that it can be glanced at discreetly without the patient's noticing.
- Take notes on the clipboard scratch paper in an *abbreviated form, quickly written*. If you are taking a long time to write out copious notes and seem to be more focused on the clipboard than on listening to the patient's responses, credit may be withheld.
- In any performance situation, one may be extremely self-conscious and lose focus on the patient. Your attention should be on a) the interesting *medical case*, trying to figure out what the patient has, and b) the *feelings and responses*, both verbal and physical, of the patient as a human being. If the patient senses that you are truly paying *keen attention* to him or her, credit will be granted.

6. **Conveyed a respectful and nonjudgmental attitude**

   - Your *body language* should convey an attitude of *openness and receptivity* to the patient. Arms held loose down to the sides show a feeling of comfort and ease in the presence of the patient. Standing or sitting in an upright yet comfortable posture communicates *self-confidence*, thus building trust. Never stand behind the patient during the history or closing because that position may suggest that you are trying to avoid making a *connection* with the patient.

   - Make sure that your *facial expressions* remain consistently nonjudgmental. For example, don't look shocked or surprised if you hear a disturbing answer; don't raise eyebrows or frown.

   - Use phrases like "okay" and "all right" rather than "good". Again, these responses establish an *open, safe atmosphere* that encourages the patient to be honest with you. Reserve all patient education for the very end of the encounter.

7. **Used appropriate draping technique**

   - The drape sheet is folded on the stool in every examining room. Just after introducing yourself and starting the interview, reach for the drape, unfold it halfway, and place it immediately on the patient from the waist down, whether the patient is lying or sitting. The bare legs are covered up, helping make the *patient feel less vulnerable*. Strictly speaking, credit will be given as long as you drape the patient no later than the beginning of the physical exam. However, it is preferable to do so at the beginning of the history to show greater respect for the patient's privacy.

   - *Ask permission* or let the patient know that you are going to untie the gown or move the drape.

   - For any maneuver, *as little of the body should be exposed as necessary*. For instance, to auscultate the heart, do not raise the gown up from the waist, exposing the entire torso. Rather, lower the gown from the top, exposing only the upper chest and shoulders.

   - As soon as you have completed examining a particular section of the body, the gown or drape should be *replaced without delay*.

8. **Used transitional phrases and references**

   Transitional statements should be made four or five times throughout the encounter. They show evidence of *orderly thinking* while *involving the patient more actively* in the process of gathering information. Appropriate places for transitional sentences are between the history of present illness and past medical history; before the sexual history; before asking about tobacco, alcohol, and recreational drug use; and before the physical exam and before the closure.

9. **Expressed empathy (reflected patient's feelings) and made appropriate reassurances**

   - You should come across as deeply concerned about the patient's well-being. One way you can show concern is by attending to the patient's *physical comfort*, by extending the leg rest when the patient lies back and then pushing it back in when the patient is sitting up; pulling out the foot step whenever the patient needs to step down onto the floor; and *supporting the patient* by holding the arm or back when lying down or sitting up. If the patient seems to be in extreme pain, say, "You look like you're in pain. Is there anything I can do to help you feel more comfortable right now?"

   - Likewise, you show true concern by responding *empathically* to the emotional states of the patient. If a sensitive issue has arisen and the patient is hesitating or perhaps beginning to cry, pause in silence for two or three full seconds, allowing the patient to process feelings, then say something like, "You must be going through a lot," or "This must have been a difficult time for you. Can you tell me about it?" A general tone of *kindness and sensitivity* should be maintained.

Tip

Practice these skills in front of a mirror. Also, interview a colleague or friend and ask for feedback about your skills of nonverbal communication.

- The *patient's beliefs* should not be denied, even if they seem implausible to the physician. If the patient says, "Oh, it's only a vitamin B deficiency," you can respond, "That's one possibility. I'd also like to check some other possibilities."

- Some suggested sentence beginnings for expressing empathy may include: "I imagine you must be…"; "It seems like you may be…"; "This must be…"; and "I'm aware it can be…"

- SPs are supposed to ask a *challenging question*, such as: "Does this mean I'm going to die/to be hospitalized/to have surgery?" The physician's response to these questions should generally be something like this: "Ms. Jones, I need to be very systematic and careful. So let's take one step at a time. First I need to have you take some blood and urine tests and some x-rays (*whichever are appropriate for the case*). Then after I study the results, I'll be able to give you a definite diagnosis and explain your options for treatment. You and I will sit down at that time and go over everything in detail. Okay?"

- It is *inappropriate* to assure a patient that he or she will get well or be cured, or to say that the condition is not serious or not to worry. It is *appropriate* to reassure the patient that you will be extremely thorough, that you will help the patient get through this difficult time, and that they are in a safe place with an excellent medical staff.

10. **Gave patient time to think and to answer without interrupting**

   - Wait in silence for the patient to think or to process feelings. The patient should *not feel rushed*. If you quickly repeat a question before the patient has had time to respond, the patient may feel that you really don't care whether the response is accurate, just that it is given rapidly.

   - Likewise, the patient's answers should not be cut off. *Quietly wait* for the patient to complete each answer. *Don't fill in words* for the patient; the answer should be in his or her own words.

11. **Asked a few open-ended questions**

   Open-ended questions (e.g., those that *require a sentence or two* describing something in the *patient's own words*) are important in eliciting information from the patient. Approximately three or four times during the entire history, ask an open-ended question.

12. **Used nonleading questions**

   The questions should be stated in a neutral manner to avoid leading the patient into answering in a way that may not be completely truthful. Generally, this kind of neutrality is achieved by using the *affirmative mode*, rather than the negative: "Mr. Brown, have you ever smoked?" instead of "You don't smoke, do you?" A neutral, *nonleading tone* encourages the patient to answer in a candid way.

13. **Asked one question at a time**

   Again, only one question should be asked at a time. Ask the question, then *pause and wait* for an answer before going on to the next item. Too often, physicians run questions together in a list. Asking questions without giving the patient an opportunity to answer interferes with clear communication.

14. **Used lay language (volunteered information if used medical terminology)**

   The appropriate language is that which any speaker of English can understand, *with or without a specialized education*. If you accidentally use a technical or medical term, immediately explain what it means in simple, straightforward language. The SP will give credit on this basis. If you use medical terminology without explaining, or if the patient has to ask what a term means, credit will not be given.

Note

Asking the patients what they believe is causing their symptoms provides the clinician with premier information about the meanings patients attach to symptoms and also what they fear.

KAPLAN
medical

15. **Effectively listened and paraphrased information given by patient throughout the encounter**

    All through the encounter, you should *reflect* what the patient has just said, by either briefly repeating or rephrasing the patient's key words. In this way, the patient knows that you are *listening* and are getting the *information correct*. Paraphrasing gives the patient the chance to correct any wrong information.

16. **Was connected and purposeful during the physical examination**

    - You are expected to interact with an SP as you would any real patient you might see with similar problems in the office, clinic, or emergency room. Examinees should demonstrate purposeful exploration of relevant components of the physical exam, with correct physical diagnostic maneuvers. (You will not have time to do a complete physical examination on every patient, which would not be necessary anyway.) Being aware and attentive to patient discomfort and modesty is important.

    - Case presentations are developed to simulate real clinical scenarios with more than one diagnostic possibility.

17. **Summarized significant information during closing, and discussed diagnostic tests**

    - Before sharing your diagnostic impression, you should summarize four to five important points from the history and physical exam that have led to your preliminary conclusions.

    - By the end of the encounter, the patient should know *what to do next*. In most cases, this is accomplished simply by the physician's stating which *general tests* need to be run, such as blood test, urine test, or x-rays.

    - *Technical terminology should not be used* in specifying lab work. Again, if you use a technical term, clarify what the test comprises before the patient has to ask what it is. When a physician uses technical terms, a distance is wedged between the physician and patient because the patient does not know the meaning of the sophisticated terms and is thus left feeling minimized and ignorant. Never *undermine a positive rapport* with the patient by showing off your technical expertise by using medical jargon.

    - In addition, for psychiatric cases, such as depression, the next step for the patient often includes knowing about *support* available in the hospital or community, such as counseling or peer support groups.

    - If the patient says he or she can't afford the tests, state that the *social services office* can work with the patient to identify *financial or other resources* available in the community.

18. **Placed patient at ease and communicated information without alarming patient**

    - Talk with the patient during the physical exam to *reduce the patient's anxiety and increase cooperation*. As you are about to perform the various maneuvers, tell the patient what you are going to do (e.g., look in the ears) and possibly why (e.g., to see whether there is any redness). If you proceed through the physical exam without speaking to the patient, no credit will be given for this item.

    - You are supposed to share your *diagnostic impression* with the patient so that he or she should have some concept of what may be wrong by the time the encounter is complete. Certainly, an *organ or body system* could be named (heart, lungs, liver, immune system) or a *general condition* could be stated (infection, virus, blockage, inflammation). Beyond that, it is expected that you specify *one of your possible differentials* of the diagnosis, but *not a definitive diagnosis*. For the purposes of the Step 2 CS exam, you are presumed to be practicing medicine *under supervision* and so would not be authorized to state a single, definitive diagnosis at this stage of the patient encounter.

    - If a medical term, such as a name of a disease, must be used, immediately explain the nature of the disease to the patient in *simple, straightforward language*. Credit is given for this use of medical terminology. However, if you do not explain the term before the patient has to ask what it means, credit would not be given.

19. Asked if patient had questions, and then answered promptly

- Always ask whether the patient has any questions before you leave, and answer them briefly in a clear, plain, and reassuring manner.

- By the time you leave the examining room, the patient should feel adequately informed, supported, and ready to take the next step. Any worries or concerns should have been addressed in a way that is appropriate at this stage of patient management.

Spoken English Proficiency

No one can alter his or her accent in a few days or weeks. However, certain techniques can be used to increase comprehensibility from low (very difficult to understand), to medium (fairly easy to understand), to high (very easy to understand). The SP does not rate you on whether you have an accent, but on how easy it is to follow your spoken English. For example, some native English speakers are difficult to follow because they talk too fast and use a choppy sentence organization.

Remembering that the Step 2 CS is primarily a test of effective communication skills, make every effort to speak clearly enough that the patient can understand what you are saying. The following are some recommendations for more effective spoken language:

- Speak more slowly than you usually do in casual conversation.

- Questions and sentences should be relatively short and to the point.

- The phrasing used should not require any interpretation on the part of the patient. For instance, the question, "Do you practice safe sex?" should be replaced by "Do you use condoms?"

- Words should be short and nontechnical. If the patient shows any sign of confusion or misunderstanding, quickly rephrase the question or statement in a simpler, more straightforward way. Recovery strategies of this kind are an integral part of effective communication.

THE CHALLENGING PATIENT

During the Step 2 CS examination, you will be presented with interpersonal challenges in addition to the clinical aspects of the case. Patient challenges include, but are not limited to, anxiety, depression, requests for immediate relief of pain, verbosity, decreased hearing or vision, an unclear reason for the visit, and emotional reactions, e.g., crying, laughing, or anger.

How to Handle Specific Patient Challenges

"I'm in pain. Can I have something for this pain?"

The best way to handle this situation is to acknowledge patients' pain and suffering and explain that you will certainly get them something for the pain after you have carefully evaluated them and if it is safe to do so. Remember that in certain cases, i.e., abdominal pain, it may actually be contraindicated to give pain medication.

The patient doesn't want to cooperate with the physical exam.

Often, if the patient is in severe pain, he or she does not want to move around for the physical examination. First, do as much of the exam as you can with the patient in his or her preferred position. For example, you could certainly do most of an ENT exam with the patient lying back—he or she does not need to sit up. There are certain parts of the exam where the patient really does need to move. For example, you cannot do an abdominal examination with the patient lying on his side; he must try to lie flat on his back. If the patient refuses to move, you need to explain how important it is to do the exam correctly and ask him to move. For a nicer touch, offer to help him to move into the necessary position. If the patient still refuses to move after all this, simply move on and document in your note.

"Doctor, am I going to die?"

This challenging question may occur on the Step 2 CS exam, and there are many ways to handle it. You need to balance your answers so they neither alarm the patient nor give false reassurances. A good way to do this is to say something like, "Your condition may be serious, but until I get more of the tests back, I can't really tell you more than that. You should also know that we have an excellent team of doctors and nurses to help you through this."

"What kind of test is that? Will it hurt?"

Remember that every time you tell a patient that you want to do a test, you should describe the test in lay terms and let him or her know if it will hurt. For example, an EKG is a heart monitor test that doesn't hurt. Of course, some tests really do hurt, i.e., lumbar puncture, but the best way to say that is, "You may experience some discomfort."

The emotional patient

A patient may be angry because of a long wait before entering the examination room or because other clinicians have been unable to solve his or her problem. Be prepared to manage these clinical challenges by identifying them and then discussing them with the patient: "Ms. Violet, I can see you are angry. Can I help?"; "Mr. Green, I know you are depressed about your symptoms and I want to help you feel better"; and "Ms. Tine, here is a box of tissues. Are you able to tell me why you are crying?"

The verbose patient

Redirecting the verbose patient to the essence of the history requires patience and finesse. At the right moment, gently interrupt and guide the patient back to a discussion of symptoms. Under these circumstances, closed-ended questions are a great way to refocus the discussion.

The reluctant patient

How will a patient present with an unclear agenda? One example is the patient who is visiting you because the appointment was made by another person without clarification about the reason for concern (i.e., an adolescent who states her mother made the appointment for a "checkup"). When faced with this challenge, begin with an open-ended question: "Why is your mother concerned?" or "Now that you are here, how can I help you?" The clinician needs to be patient and kind.

ENDING THE INTERVIEW

The time available for the entire counseling component of the 15-minute patient encounter is about 2 to 4 minutes. Present the most likely diagnosis with one or two other possibilities, then describe the diagnostic tests that will provide the information to complete the evaluation. Prior to exiting, ask the patient if more information is needed or if there are unanswered questions. Do not shake hands unless the patient offers first.

IN SUMMARY

Closing the Encounter

- Briefly summarize what you have heard in the history or found in the physical exam.
- Briefly explain your most likely differential diagnosis.
- Explain the testing you need to do in order to arrive at a conclusion.
- Reserve management discussions "until we are sure what the problem is."
- Avoid offering pain meds during the encounter.
- Avoid alarming the patient; be careful and sensitive in the way you explain the possible diagnosis. However, you must let the patient know what you are considering. Say that you "promise" to consider such and such, if it is something frightening like a tumor.
- Ask if the patient has any questions. Answer each question clearly with reassurance.
- Reassure the patient that you will do everything you can to help.
- Shake patient's hand—if offered—and say, "I'll follow up with you as soon as I receive the results."
- Leave the room.

Chapter Three: **Focused Medical History**

THE MEDICAL INTERVIEW

During the Step 2 CS examination, your primary task is to generate differential diagnoses and an appropriate diagnostic workup based on the information provided to you: the patient's symptoms, thoughtful history taking, and performing a focused physical examination. The note should clearly reflect this process, thereby placing emphasis on primary data elicited during the patient interaction and not on the results of tests or the opinions of consultants.

Introductory (Doorway) Information

Preliminary (introductory) information about the patient will be available on the doorway of the examination room (additional copies are placed inside the room and at the site where you'll write your note). It provides the name, age, and sex of the patient and the initial chief concern or complaint. Also listed will be the vital signs—temperature in degrees Fahrenheit and Centigrade, blood pressure, and heart and respiratory rates. Using these facts, it is important to begin generating hypotheses that will lead to the correct diagnosis. This process will help you save time by narrowing your initial questioning to the most likely possibilities. Remember to be a good listener; you still may have to recast your initial assumptions following the patient's responses.

Note

There will likely be only one main clinical problem rather than multiple ones because of the short encounter and the time needed by the SP to evaluate your performance of the history, physical examination, and communication skills.

CLINICAL EXERCISE 1

Below you will find examples of doorway information for seven patients. After reading and absorbing the information on them, list the three most likely hypotheses for each patient's chief concern placed in the context of the vital signs in order of likelihood (one being most likely, three being least). When you have completed this exercise, compare your lists with those found in Appendix V.

A. Ms. Edna Brown, a 74-year-old, comes to the office today because of a severe headache.

Temperature: 98.2 F, 37 C

Blood pressure: 172/92 mm Hg, right arm sitting

Pulse rate: 82/min, regular

Respiratory rate: 14/min

Hypotheses:

1._____

2._____

3._____

B. Mr. Art Muta, a 22-year-old, comes to the urgent illness clinic today because of a cough.

Temperature: 100.2 F, 38 C

Blood pressure: 124/60 mm Hg, right arm sitting

Pulse rate: 86/min, regular

Respiratory rate: 12/min

Hypotheses:

1._____

2._____

3._____

C. Mr. Sam Renee, a 78-year-old, is brought to the emergency department because of chest pain.

Temperature: 99 F, 37 C

Blood pressure: 140/96 mm Hg, right arm sitting

Pulse rate: 104/min, regular

Respiratory rate: 18/min

Hypotheses:

1._____

2._____

3._____

D. Ms. Pam Bert, a 17-year-old, comes to the office today because of severe abdominal pain.

Temperature: 102.1 F, 39 C

Blood pressure: 108/56 mm Hg, right arm sitting

Pulse rate: 110/min, regular

Respiratory rate: 16/min

Hypotheses:

1._____

2._____

3._____

E. Ms. Samantha Singer is the mother of Jennifer Singer, a 7-year-old. Ms. Singer is concerned because her daughter is having problems learning to read. Jennifer is in school today.

Hypotheses:

1._____

2._____

3._____

Note

A concern about an infant or child will be presented by a parent or guardian because it is not practical to have children as SPs. Although there will be no physical examination during this visit, components of the examination may be recommended as a "diagnostic test" in the written note.

F. Ms. Victoria Rose, a 36-year-old woman, has come to the office today with a concern of being tired all the time.

Temperature: 98 F, 37 C

Blood pressure: 100/78 mm Hg, right arm sitting

Pulse rate: 90/min, regular

Respiratory rate: 11/min

Hypotheses:

1. _____

2. _____

3. _____

G. Mr. Ira Ring, a 38-year-old, presents to your office because of pain in his lower back.

Temperature: 98.6 F, 37 C

Blood pressure: 138/88 mm Hg, right arm sitting

Pulse rate: 72/min

Respiratory rate: 12/min

Hypotheses:

1. _____

2. _____

3. _____

PERFORMING THE FOCUSED HISTORY

Thoughtfully apportion your time to achieve a sharply focused interview. The key is the active process of generating hypotheses, i.e., rapidly working toward preparing an insightful differential diagnosis of the patient's clinical problem. You are continuing the reasoning you began when you read the chief concern on the doorway. Explore possibilities using clear open- and close-ended questions to elicit the history of the present illness (*see* Table 3-1).

Table 3-1. History of the Present Illness (HPI)

> **S**ite of the symptom (e.g., on the back between the shoulder blades)
>
> **I**ntensity/quantity of the symptom (e.g., 7/10 on a scale from 1 to 10; 1 tsp of blood)
>
> **Q**uality of the symptom (e.g., stabbing pain)
>
> **O**nset of the symptom (e.g., started after a sudden stop while driving), precipitating factors, timing, and course duration
>
> **R**adiation (e.g., pain travels down back)
>
> **A**ggravating factors that make the symptoms worse
>
> **A**lleviating factors that make the symptoms better
>
> **A**ssociated manifestations (e.g., fever, shortness of breath, headache)

These parameters serve as an invaluable guide in organizing a description of the present illness. Although some diseases do not manifest all of these dimensions, their use in history taking is very reliable.

A careful clinician's HPI includes the absence of relevant symptoms (pertinent negatives), along with the described symptoms. Negative information is as important as the positive to enable accurate formulation and testing of hypotheses.

Site

Patients generally refer to bodily location in lay terms, rather than in technical ones, and broadly rather than specifically, e.g., "headache," "stomachache," or "backache." It is up to the clinician to localize the exact region with precision, and it is helpful to have the patient identify the area by pointing.

Intensity/Quantity

Questions related to quantity include frequency, size, volume, and number. "How many times did you vomit today?" "How often does the stomach pain occur?" A patient may say that he's been coughing up "a lot of blood," when it turns out to be less than a teaspoon. The intensity of a symptom may be ascertained by asking the patient to use the 1 to 10 scale. The degree of functional impairment is quantified by getting specific details about what a patient can do and for how long.

Quality

Begin by generally asking what the symptom feels like. If vague terms are used, ask the patient to relate it to some previous similar pain. It is often necessary for the clinician to ask leading questions, e.g., "Is the pain sharp or dull? Is the nausea constant or intermittent?"

**Kaplan Medical's
HPI Mnemonic**

SIQOR AAA
(pronounced "sicker AAA")

The HPI questions related to these dimensions do not need to be asked in this particular order, but rather as they naturally present for each case.

Step 2 CS Strategy

The focused physical examination required for the Step 2 CS examination may begin during the HPI by being alert to identifying visible abnormal physical findings.

Note

It is impossible to overstate the importance of scrupulous attention to detail when dating the onset of symptoms and following the chronology of an illness.

Onset

Dates and times when symptoms first began are consistently the most reliable descriptors with which to develop the present illness. Referring to the very first time a symptom appeared is most revealing. Patients may minimize early prodromal symptoms that seem unimportant to them but which are very critical diagnostically. Always establish the last time when a patient felt in a normal state of health.

Establishing the setting in which the patient's illness has developed and the location and time when symptoms occur helps the clinician to add precision to the HPI that is required as hypotheses are tested. Setting refers to where and when symptoms occur. The frenzy of an office at tax preparation time is obviously relevant when an accountant comes in with burning epigastric pain. For someone who has diarrhea, a recent trip abroad is relevant. Dyspnea occurring in the early morning hours is a clue to the presence of congestive heart failure.

Radiation

Questions related to depth are useful because patients often can tell, in a general way, whether the pain feels on the surface of their body or deep within. Radiation is an essential dimension to explore, but rather than use the clinical term "radiation," ask where the symptom moves to, e.g., through to the back? down into the left arm? up to the jaw?

Aggravating factors

Questions that elucidate what makes symptoms worse give clues to the etiology and severity. Common factors include position, activity level, exertion, relation to food, time of day, and medication use.

Alleviating factors

Questions that elucidate what makes symptoms better give clues to the etiology and severity. Common factors include position, activity level, exertion, relation to food, time of day, and medication use.

Associated manifestations

Probe for other symptoms the patient has had by testing the range of symptoms associated with the hypotheses generated. For example, it is necessary to ask a young woman with joint pain about rashes and unexplained fever if systemic lupus erythematosus is a consideration. Asking for "any other symptoms" in a general way during the Step 2 CS examination will have a low yield because the standardized patients are trained to respond with a vague answer.

OTHER COMPONENTS OF THE PATIENT'S HISTORY

During the Step 2 CS examination, the focus is on the history of the present illness (HPI). Other aspects of the history should be incorporated if they have relevance to the HPI. Testing your hypotheses by asking about the characteristics of the present illness will disclose those aspects of the past medical history, family history, social history, and review of systems that should be asked and recorded in the note.

The following table may assist you in obtaining most of the components of the past medical history.

Kaplan Medical's PMH Mnemonic

Table 3-2. Past Medical History (PMH)*

Previous experience of chief complaint	P
Allergies (to foods, medicines, plants, animals)	A
Medicines	M
History of hospitalization/surgery/illness/injury or accident	H
Review of systems	R
Family history (focus on problems similar to patient's chief complaint and HPI, as well as other serious illnesses or conditions in general)	F
OB/GYN (e.g., last menstrual period, gravida, para, abortions, infections)	O
Sexual history (sexually active, number of partners, male/female/both, condom use, STDs)	S
Social history (work situation, home life, environmental changes, smoking, alcohol, recreational drugs)	S

*Use these as needed, depending on their relevance to the HPI.

For a more general, in-depth review addressing specific components of the patient history, see Appendix III.

CLINICAL EXERCISE 2

We will now conduct the medical interview of the patients presented and discussed in Clinical Exercise 1. The doorway information is repeated. Assume you have entered the patient's room, introduced yourself, and properly covered the lower limbs with the draping sheet. With each clinical example, there are three blank areas to write questions you would ask for each aspect of the HPI noted in Table 3-1. When you have completed this exercise, compare your responses with those found in Appendix V.

> **A.** Ms. Edna Brown, a 74-year-old, comes to the office today because of a severe headache.
>
> Temperature: 98.2 F, 37 C
>
> Blood pressure: 172/92 mm Hg, right arm sitting
>
> Pulse rate: 82/min, regular
>
> Respiratory rate: 14/min

Remember

Kaplan Medical Mnemonic
SIQOR AAA

Site:

1._____

Intensity/Quantity:

1._____

2._____

3._____

Quality:

1._____

2._____

3._____

Onset:

1._____

2._____

3._____

4._____

5._____

6._____

Radiation:

1._____

Aggravating or Alleviating factors:

1._____

2._____

3._____

Associated manifestations:

1._____

2._____

3._____

B. Mr. Art Muta, a 22-year-old, comes to urgent illness clinic today because of a cough.

Temperature: 100.2 F, 38 C

Blood pressure: 124/60 mm Hg, right arm sitting

Pulse rate: 86/min, regular

Respiratory rate: 12/min

Site:

1._____

Intensity/Quantity:

1._____

2._____

3._____

Quality:

1._____

2._____

3._____

Onset:

1._____

2._____

3._____

4._____

5._____

6._____

Radiation:

1._____

Aggravating or Alleviating factors:

1._____

2._____

3._____

Associated manifestations:

1._____

2._____

3._____

4._____

C. Mr. Sam Renee, a 78-year-old, is brought to the emergency department because of chest pain.

Temperature: 99 F, 37 C

Blood pressure: 140/96 mm Hg, right arm sitting

Pulse rate: 104/min, regular

Respiratory rate: 18/min

Site:

1._____

2._____

Intensity/Quantity:

1._____

2._____

3._____

Quality:

1._____

2._____

3._____

Onset:

1._____

2._____

3._____

4._____

5._____

6._____

Radiation:

1._____

Aggravating or Alleviating factors:

1._____

2._____

3._____

Associated manifestations:

1._____

2._____

3._____

D.   Ms. Pam Bert, a 17-year-old, comes to the office today because of severe abdominal pain.

Temperature: 102.1 F, 39 C

Blood pressure: 108/56 mm Hg, right arm sitting

Pulse rate: 110/min, regular

Respiratory rate: 16/min

Site:

1._____

2._____

Intensity/Quantity:

1._____

2._____

3._____

Quality:

1._____

2._____

3._____

Onset:

1._____

2._____

3._____

4._____

5._____

6._____

Radiation:

1._____

Aggravating or Alleviating factors:

1._____

2._____

3._____

Associated manifestations:

1._____

2._____

3._____

E.   Ms. Samantha Singer is the mother of Jennifer Singer, a 7-year-old. Ms. Singer is concerned because her daughter is having problems learning to read. Jennifer is in school today.

Site:

1._____

2._____

3._____

Intensity/Quantity:

1._____

2._____

3._____

Quality:

1._____

2._____

3._____

Onset:

1._____

2._____

3._____

4._____

5._____

6._____

Aggravating or Alleviating factors:

1._____

2._____

3._____

F.   Ms. Victoria Rose, a 36-year-old woman, has come to the office today
        with a concern of being tired all the time.

Temperature: 98 F, 37 C

Blood pressure: 100/78 mm Hg, right arm sitting

Pulse rate: 90/min, regular

Respiratory rate: 11/min

Site:

1._____

2._____

3._____

Intensity/Quantity:

1._____

2._____

3._____

Quality:

1._____

2._____

3._____

Onset:

1._____

2._____

3._____

4._____

5._____

6._____

Aggravating or Alleviating factors:

1._____

2._____

3._____

Associated manifestations:

1._____

2._____

3._____

G. Mr. Ira Ring, a 38-year-old, presents to your office because of pain in his lower back.

Temperature: 98.6 F, 37 C

Blood pressure: 138/88 mm Hg, right arm sitting

Pulse rate: 72/min

Respiratory rate: 12/min

Site:

1._____

2._____

Intensity/Quantity:

1._____

2._____

3._____

Quality:

1._____

2._____

3._____

Onset:

1._____

2._____

3._____

4._____

5._____

6._____

Radiation:

1._____

Aggravating or Alleviating factors:

1._____

2._____

3._____

Associated manifestations:

1._____

2._____

3._____

Chapter Four: **Focused Physical Exam**

GENERAL POINTS

To perform a targeted physical examination, you must have a well-considered differential diagnosis and knowledge of which physical findings would be expected for each condition included in the differential. Because of the time constraint imposed by the Step 2 CS, keeping the exam focused is crucial.

- Standardized patients (SPs) are diligently trained to simulate the illness being portrayed. Physical findings can be imitated and enhanced by the application of stage makeup. Actors can be found who have actual abnormalities that can be placed into the setting of the case. A person with a known cardiac murmur can reliably simulate a patient with infective endocarditis. *Therefore, consider all detected abnormalities as real.*

- At the appropriate time, tell the patient that you are now going to conduct the examination, and wash your hands before proceeding.

- Then begin in a logical manner, moving from head to feet. As you examine a region, describe what you are doing to the patient; for example, "I am examining your ears to see if you have an infection."

- Drape the patient with care and never examine a patient through clothing. Politely ask the patient's assistance whenever clothing needs to be moved to provide the correct exposure. Breast, pelvic, rectal, or genital exams are not permitted. (Indicate their necessity in the diagnostic workup section of the patient note.) To examine the heart in a woman, listen to all areas of the heart around the patient's bra. It is permissible to place the stethoscope down between the breasts to continue listening. If you need to auscultate or palpate for the PMI, ask the patient to please hold her breast up.

- Write information on the blue sheet: identified physical findings, new information provided by the patient, and differential diagnoses.

- If the patient is in severe pain and refusing an examination, ask again gently and only once. Then say something such as, "I know you are in pain. This exam will help me to understand what is causing it." If necessary, assist the patient into exam position and say, "I know you are in pain, but let me help you. I'll do this as quickly as possible. I'll let you know exactly what I'm going to do before I do it."

- Continue to ask questions as needed about the history of the present illness during the focused physical examination. For example, if unexpected petechiae are noted, ask the patient when they first appeared. Continually interweaving the history and physical examination increases the accurate identification of key information and can more accurately modify the initially generated hypotheses.

Timing and Scoring

You should allow between *4 and 6 minutes* to perform the physical exam. Remember, the Step 2 CS physical, like the history, is scored by the SP on a checklist. Points are gained by *correctly* examining what is on the checklist for the specific presenting condition. If something on the checklist is not done, no points will be given for that item. Conversely, if a part of the body is examined and that item is not on the list, no extra points will be given. Therefore, your main objective is to *thoroughly* examine the target area, and then use the remaining time to examine other areas related to your differential. For example:

A 73-year-old male hypertensive smoker presents with left-sided chest pain, nausea, diaphoresis, and palpitations.

Differential diagnosis

*   Angina
*   MI
*   Costochondritis
*   Pneumonia
*   Pneumothorax

Sample physical exam checklist

*   Washed hands prior to exam
*   Palpated the PMI
*   Inspected for JVD
*   Checked pulses (at least two places)
*   Palpated for chest wall tenderness
*   Auscultated heart at apex and base, sitting/supine
*   Auscultated lungs front and back, side to side, two levels

In this obviously cardiac case, the cardiac exam was thorough and complete. However, because pulmonary diseases were also in the differential diagnosis, auscultation of the lungs would be expected on this physical exam checklist. If you had performed a more thorough pulmonary exam in this case, no points would have been deducted, but none gained either. So, it is important to perform a very thorough examination of the main *target areas* to gain as many points as possible. Then move to related systems as time permits.

Sometimes, the two leading diagnoses in your differential may be from different systems (e.g., CHF versus pneumonia). In such a case, perform as complete an exam of each system as time permits. Remember, too, that you are expected to discuss the case with the SP at the end of the encounter, so you must leave 1 to 2 minutes for closure.

CLINICAL EXERCISE 3

Focused Physical Examination

Preparation for the focused physical examination component of the Step 2 CS examination requires thoughtful practice. Although you may have listed initial hypotheses (differential diagnoses) that are different from those seen in this exercise, please list the region(s) to be examined based on the three hypotheses below. Skin must be examined as you examine a region. When you have completed this exercise, compare your notes with the answers found in Appendix V.

A. Ms. Edna Brown, a 74-year-old, comes to the office today because of a severe headache.

Temperature: 98.2 F, 37 C

Blood pressure: 172/92 mm Hg, right arm sitting

Pulse rate: 82/min, regular

Respiratory rate: 14/min

Hypotheses:

1. Muscle contraction (tension) headache

2. Migraine headache

3. Intracerebral or subarachnoid hemorrhage

Region(s) to be examined:

_____

_____

_____

B.   Mr. Art Muta, a 22-year-old, comes to urgent illness clinic today because of a cough.

Temperature: 100.2 F, 38 C

Blood pressure: 124/60 mm Hg, right arm sitting

Pulse rate: 86/min, regular

Respiratory rate: 12/min

Hypotheses:

1.   Upper respiratory infection
2.   Acute bronchitis
3.   Community-acquired pneumonia

Region(s) to be examined:

_____

_____

_____

C.   Mr. Sam Renee, a 78-year-old, is brought to the emergency department because of chest pain.

Temperature: 99 F, 37 C

Blood pressure: 140/96 mm Hg, right arm sitting

Pulse rate: 104/min, regular

Respiratory rate: 18/min

Hypotheses:

1.   Acute coronary syndrome: unstable angina or acute myocardial infarction
2.   Acute infectious pleuritis, possible initial presentation of *S. pneumoniae* pneumonia
3.   Musculoskeletal chest pain

Region(s) to be examined:

_____

_____

_____

D. Ms. Pam Bert, a 17-year-old, comes to the office today because of severe abdominal pain.

Temperature: 102.1 F, 39 C

Blood pressure: 108/56 mm Hg, right arm sitting

Pulse rate: 110/min, regular

Respiratory rate: 16/min

Hypotheses:
1. Acute appendicitis
2. Nonspecific gastroenteritis
3. Rupture of a tubal pregnancy

Region(s) to be examined:

_____

_____

_____

E. Ms. Samantha Singer is the mother of Jennifer Singer, a 7-year-old. Ms. Singer is concerned because her daughter is having problems learning to read. Jennifer is in school today.

Hypotheses:
1. Learning disability
2. Visual or auditory impairment
3. Behavioral disorder

In this case the child is not present; request the physical examination as a "diagnostic test" when the note is written.

F.   Ms. Victoria Rose, a 36-year-old woman, has come to the office today with a concern of being tired all the time.

Temperature: 98 F, 37 C

Blood pressure: 100/78 mm Hg, right arm sitting

Pulse rate: 90/min, regular

Respiratory rate: 11/min

Hypotheses:

1.   Depression/anxiety
2.   Anemia, likely iron-deficiency
3.   Hypothyroidism

Region(s) to be examined:

_____

_____

_____

G.   Mr. Ira Ring, a 38-year-old, presents to your office because of pain in his lower back.

Temperature: 98.6 F, 37 C

Blood pressure: 138/88 mm Hg, right arm sitting

Pulse rate: 72/min

Respiratory rate: 12/min

Hypotheses:

1.   Acute or chronic musculoskeletal pain, i.e., lumbosacral strain
2.   Intervertebral disk disease
3.   Inflammatory arthropathy, e.g., ankylosing spondylitis

Region(s) to be examined:

_____

_____

_____

FOCUSED EXAMS BY SYSTEM

Head, Eyes, Ears, Nose and Throat (HEENT) Exam

When to do an HEENT exam

Complaints of:

1) Headache

2) Head trauma

3) Ocular problems (visual disturbance, eye pain)

4) Ear problems (tinnitus, vertigo, hearing loss)

5) Nasal problems (rhinorrhea, epistaxis, sinus pain)

6) Pharyngitis, voice changes, jaw pain

How to do the exam

1) Head

- Inspect for trauma, scars, abnormalities

2) Eyes

- Inspect sclera/conjunctiva for color, irritation; pupils for symmetry, reactivity, extraocular movements
- Inspect visual acuity with Snellen eye chart if patient has visual complaint
- How to use the *ophthalmoscope* for funduscopic abnormalities
    1) Make sure the unit is turned on
    2) Remove from holder
    3) Shine light on hand
    4) Adjust lenses
    5) Check light reflexes
    6) Ask patient to stare at point on wall
    7) Come in from side—use your right eye for patient's right eye and hold instrument in right hand; use left eye for patient's left eye and hold instrument in left hand

3) Ears

- Inspect external ear for abnormalities
- Palpate ear, mastoid area
- How to use the otoscope for tympanic membrane and ear canal
    1) Turn light on
    2) Remove from holder
    3) Put on a *new* speculum
    4) Palpate ear for tenderness
    5) Pull pinna up, out, and back
    6) Inspect canal and tympanic membrane
- Perform Weber and Rinne test if complaint of hearing loss

Rinne

    1) Place vibrating tuning fork on mastoid process

    2) When patient no longer hears it, move to external ear

Weber

    1) Place vibrating tuning fork on center of forehead

    2) Check if sound is equal in both ears

4) Nose

- Inspect external nose
- Palpate nose and sinuses
- Inspect nasal turbinates with light source

5) Throat

- Inspect with light source
- Check for movement of palate
- Examine floor of mouth
- Examine posterior oral cavity using tongue depressor

Neurologic Exam

When to do a neurologic exam

Complaints of:

1) Headache
2) Dizziness, vertigo
3) Balance problems
4) Visual disturbances
5) Muscle weakness
6) Psychiatric problems
7) Sensory problems; numbness or tingling
8) Memory problems

How to do the exam

1) Mental status

- Orientation (level of consciousness, orientation to person, place, and time)
- Concentration (serial sevens or "world")
- Memory (remember three things); ask to repeat after a few minutes

2) Cranial nerves

- I: Not formally tested
- II: Vision (use the Snellen chart to check for activity, then check visual fields)
- III, IV, VI: Extraocular movements
- V: Sensation on face (three areas), clench teeth
- VII: Bare teeth, lift brow

- • IX, X: Gag or check palate for symmetrical movement
- • XI: Trapezius or sternocleidomastoid strength (shrug shoulders)
- • XII: Stick out tongue

3) Motor
- • Arms: Pull in, push out
- • Wrists: Pull up, push down
- • Hands: Fingers spread apart
- • Legs: Kick out, pull in
- • Ankles: Push on the gas

4) Reflexes (*see* Figure 4-1)
- • Biceps
- • Triceps
- • Brachioradialis
- • Patellar
- • Achilles
- • Babinski

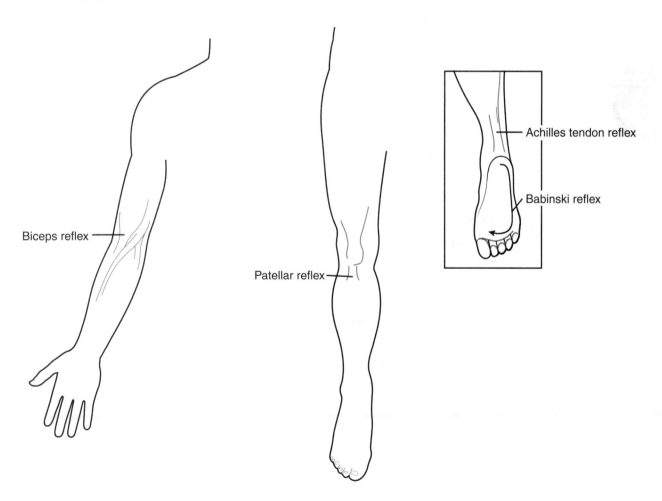

Figure 4-1. Eliciting the Reflexes

KAPLAN
medical

5) Sensory
- Tell patient to close eyes
- Demonstrate sharp/dull
- Test all possible affected areas
- Repeat with light touch

6) Cerebellar
- Finger to nose
- Romberg sign—patient stands with feet together, arms out, palms up, eyes closed and head back; positive if patient loses balance
- Heel to shin
- Gait—patient walks across room; may try tandem gait also

7) Specific tests
- Kernig (if meningitis suspected)—patient lying on table with knees flexed; straighten leg out to see if patient has pain
- Brudzinski (if meningitis suspected)—bring chin to chest
- Babinski—stroke lateral edge to plantar surface of foot

Pulmonary Exam

When to do a pulmonary exam

Complaints of:

1) Cough
2) Shortness of breath
3) Wheezing
4) Chest pain
5) Upper respiratory infection symptoms

How to do the exam

1) Inspect
- Respiratory rate
- Respiratory pattern
- Hands (for cyanosis or clubbing)

2) Palpate
- Chest wall tenderness
- Chest excursion
- Tactile fremitus (use lateral surface of hand, ask patient to say "99")

3) Percuss
- Front of chest
- Back of chest

Remember

Palpation and auscultation should always be done directly on the SP's skin, not through the gown.

4) Auscultate (not through gown!)

- Front of chest
- Back of chest
- Lateral chest

5) Special points

- Do not percuss or auscultate over scapulae
- Let the patient fully inhale/exhale before moving to next area
- Auscultation of the heart is strongly recommended
- Check two levels on the anterior chest; three levels posterior
- Always move from side to side

Cardiovascular Exam

When to do the cardiovascular exam

Complaints of:

1) Chest pain
2) Palpitations
3) Loss of consciousness
4) Shortness of breath
5) Pedal edema
6) Any other problem that would put a cardiac cause high in your differential diagnosis

How to do the exam

1) While the patient is sitting:

- Assess blood pressure (by having read opening scenario)
- Check pulses—auscultate carotids, then palpate; then check radial, posterior tibial, and dorsalis pedis pulses
- Check for dependent edema

2) Ask the patient to lie back on the table

- Inspect for JVD
- Palpate for PMI, heaves, thrills
- Auscultate *all four cardiac areas*

3) Ask the patient to sit up again.

- Auscultate all four cardiac areas
- Lean forward and listen at base
- Auscultate lungs
- Check for tenderness along costochondral margins

Abdominal Exam

When to do the abdominal exam

Complaints of

    1) Abdominal pain

    2) Diarrhea

    3) Vomiting

    4) Constipation

    5) Blood per rectum

    6) Jaundice

    7) UTI symptoms/hematuria

    8) Pelvic pain/suspected pregnancy

How to do the exam

    1) Inspect

      • Ask, "Have you noticed any changes in the skin on your stomach?"

    2) Auscultate

      • It is crucial to auscultate prior to palpation!

    3) Percussion

      • All four quadrants

    4) Palpate

      • It is crucial to start away from the pain and move toward it slowly.

    5) Check for rebound tenderness

      • In suspected peritonitis

      • Ask the patient, "Does it hurt more when I press in or let go?"

    6) Check for Murphy sign

      • Hand along lower edge of ribs

      • Ask patient to take deep breath in cases of suspected cholecystitis.

    7) Check the back for costovertebral angle (CVA) tenderness—gently pound over the costovertebral angle

      • In cases of suspected nephrolithiasis, pyelonephritis

    8) Don't forget:

      • If a patient needs a complete abdominal exam, he or she probably needs a rectal exam and occult blood, which you would include in your diagnostic tests section of the patient note.

Musculoskeletal Exam

When to do the musculoskeletal exam

Complaints of

    1) Joint pain, swelling, stiffness

    2) Extremity pain

    3) Decreased range of motion

4) Muscular weakness, pain

5) Fatigue, vague complaints suggestive of rheumatologic illness

How to do the exam

1) Inspect the area of concern and compare to opposite side

2) Inspect other joints for signs of abnormality

3) Palpate the area, try to elicit the pain, note swelling, edema

4) Check range of motion, assess for crepitus, limitations

5) Assess neurologic status (sensation, strength, reflexes) around the affected area

6) Assess vascular status (pulses) around affected area

7) Special points

- Wrist/hand complaints: always check nerves, other joints, tinel, phalen
  - Tinel—tap on the wrist right over the median nerve; patient has pain, tingling in median nerve distribution if positive
  - Phalen—patient puts dorsum of hands together; should have pain, tingling over median distribution if positive
- Shoulder: range of motion is critical, touch opposite shoulder
- Knee: check anterior/posterior drawer signs
- Lumbosacral spine: Check the patient's gait, reflexes, and range of motion (straight leg raise).
  - Straight leg raise—patient lies on table; left leg at ankle; patient experiences discomfort as leg is lifted

Chapter Five: **Patient Note**

OVERVIEW

This section covers how to document your patient encounter in the brief 10 minutes allowed. Your notes are graded by a health professional, and thus should be written in a way that communicates information clearly to another health care practitioner. Your notes must contain all the *pertinent positive and negative findings* from the history and physical examination, as well as a differential diagnosis and diagnostic workup. As you will see, the differential diagnosis and diagnostic workup both require you to make a list.

Blank scratch paper will be provided during each encounter. You may use this paper at your discretion to write down informal notes during the encounter. Your informal notes will be collected along with your formal patient note after you write the patient note.

Make sure to follow these suggestions:
- Patient notes may be handwritten or typed. You are graded on legibility; therefore, typing is a recommended option, providing that you can type quickly enough within the allotted 10 minutes.
- If you choose to handwrite the note, write legibly. If the reader cannot read your note, you will not get credit.
- Stay within the space allotted for each section.
- Keep your notes organized and present the information in a logical order.
- Present a reasonable list of diagnoses based on the history and physical; your workup should be designed to reduce your differential.

Although there are other acceptable ways (such as the narrative paragraph) to write a Step 2 CS patient note, we have found the list/phrase format to be an effective method. We will show you below how the format works in the different sections of the patient note.

Writing the History

The history must be presented in an organized fashion that focuses on the *relevant* positive and negative findings from the encounter. In the list/phrase format, you should list down the left column the history categories, and then write your applicable history findings in each category in a phrase format.

Begin the note with chief complaint, including the age and sex of the patient. Follow with the history of the present illness (HPI) and include all information relevant to the current problem(s) in the HPI, including past medical history, family history, habits, social history, and system review. Keep the focus sharply on the HPI and encompass positive and negative highlights.

Note

A copy of the doorway information is placed at the site where you will write the note.

Chief Complaint (CC)

This is a one sentence description of the patient's reason for the visit. Include the patient's age and sex.

History of Present Illness (HPI)

Describe the circumstances surrounding the patient's chief complaint.

- **S**ite
- **I**ntensity/Quantity
- **Q**uality
- **O**nset
- **R**adiation
- **A**ggravating factors
- **A**lleviating factors
- **A**ssociated manifestations

Past Medical History (PMI)

This is a relevant review of systems and symptoms, serious illnesses, hospitalizations, surgeries, medications, diets, weight changes, and sleep patterns.

- **P**revious event similar to the chief complaint
- **A**llergies (to foods, medicines, plants, animals)
- **M**edicines (OTC, prescriptions, vitamins, herbs)
- **H**istory of hospitalization/surgery/illnesses/trauma/injury
- **R**eview of systems
- **F**amily history (focused on problems similar to patient's CC and HPI)
- **O**B/GYN (e.g., last menstrual period [LMP], gravida, para, abortions, infections)
- **S**exual history (sexually active, number of partners, male/female/both, condom use, STDs)
- **S**ocial history (occupation, home life, environmental changes, smoking, alcohol, recreational drugs, including intravenous)

Writing the Physical Examination

List the patient's general appearance; always comment on the recorded vital signs by listing them, noting whether they are normal or abnormal. Use an outline to record the findings. Encompass positive and negative highlights.

The following are examples of what can be written for normal exams. Of course, any positive findings noted during your exam would be included as part of your write up.

Kaplan Medical Mnemonic

S
I
Q
O
R
A
A
A

Kaplan Medical Mnemonic

P
A
M
H
R
F
O
S
S

Sample documentation of a normal HEENT exam

Head: normocephalic, atraumatic

Eyes: EOM intact, PERRLA; (–) funduscopic abnormalities or papilledema

Ears: canals without abnormalities, tympanic membranes clear

Nose: nasal turbinates not congested

Throat: no tonsillar enlargement, erythema or exudates

Mouth: dentition good, (–) lesions, (–) vesicles, (–) oral thrush

Neck: supple, (–) thyroid enlargement, (–) cervical lymph nodes

Sample documentation of a normal neurologic exam

Mental status: alert, oriented ×3, good concentration

Cranial nerves: II–XII intact

Motor: strength 5 of 5 all muscle groups

DTR: 2+ intact symmetric

Sensation: intact to sharp and dull

Cerebellar: Romberg negative, finger to nose intact

Plantar reflex normal

Kernig negative, Brudzinski negative

Sample documentation of a normal respiratory exam

Breathing unlabored, rate _____

Clear to percussion & auscultation R & L

(–) Cyanosis, (–) clubbing

(–) Tenderness to palpation

(–) Dullness to percussion

(–) Rales, (–) wheezes, (–) rhonchi, (–) rubs in any lung field

Tactile fremitus within normal limits

Sample documentation of a normal cardiovascular exam

Cardiovascular: BP ____, HR ____, pulses 2+ BL

PMI nondisplaced

(–) Palpable heaves S1/S2 regular rhythm, (–) murmurs

(–) Rubs, (–) gallops, (–) JVD, (–) pedal edema

Sample documentation of a normal abdominal exam

(–) Surgical scars or skin abnormalities on inspection

Bowel sounds present (or + bowel signs)

Abd. tympanitic to percussion in all 4 quadrants, liver size normal by percussion

(–) Palpable masses, soft, nontender, nondistended to palpation

Sample documentation of a normal lumbosacral exam

No obvious deformities or signs of trauma

No spinous process or paraspinous tenderness

Range of motion normal anteriorly

Normal gait

Reflexes 2+ patellar, Achilles

Sensation intact (sharp/dull)

Sample documentation of a normal psychiatric mental status exam

Patient appears well groomed.

He is alert and oriented to person, place, and time.

Speech is fluid and goal directed.

Recent and remote memory are intact.

Attention and concentration are unimpaired as tested by serial sevens.

Mood is euthymic. Affect is consistent with mood.

The patient does not have abnormal perceptions such as hallucinations, delusions, or paranoias.

The patient denies having suicidal/homicidal ideation or intent.

Judgment/insight are intact.

Differential Diagnosis

Base the differential diagnosis on the hypotheses generated from the introductory information on the doorway, the medical interview, and physical examination. It is perfectly appropriate—and some examinees may even prefer this—to write the differential diagnosis first to ensure logical and thorough incorporation of all four sections of the written note. Try to list five differential diagnoses with the most likely one first, and use the most exacting disease terminology. Directly link a second problem with a first, e.g., AIDS with pulmonary tuberculosis. It is okay to have fewer than five options in your differential—only include realistic possibilities! Do not include long shots just to fill up space.

Diagnostic Workup

Carefully correlate diagnostic testing with the differential diagnosis you have generated. Simple, noninvasive and less expensive tests are emphasized. Omit tests of extremely limited efficacy in the scientific practice of medicine, e.g., the erythrocyte sedimentation rate or the upper gastrointestinal series. Follow the differential diagnosis by listing five diagnostic tests, and group similar tests as one, e.g., creatinine, glucose, and electrolytes, and note those with the highest probable yield first. Include invasive tests if they are crucial to the diagnosis, e.g., a lymph node biopsy of a solitary enlarged supraclavicular lymph node.

Helpful Hints

- Make sure that your differentials are derived from your history and physical findings.

- Do not include irrelevant diagnoses just to fill space.

- Make sure your diagnoses are specific, e.g., don't write "pregnancy"; instead, write "intrauterine pregnancy" or "ectopic pregnancy."

Helpful Hints

- Always write "first-line" and specific tests.

- Write your list in the order you would actually perform the tests in a clinical setting. For example, if you are considering MI, angina, and GERD as likely diagnoses, first consider CPK-MB, troponin. Then consider an EKG. Finally, consider EGD if all previous tests were negative.

- Write all related tests on one line, e.g., all blood tests or all x-rays should be written on the same line.

- Do *not* order treatment, hospitalization, referrals, or consultations (these are not diagnostic).

- Breast, rectal, pelvic, genital, and corneal reflex exams cannot be performed on SPs during the encounter; if indicated, these procedures should be listed in this section. However, these exams are still clinically important, and you should be comfortable and adept at performing them.

GENERIC PATIENT NOTE TEMPLATE

Patient Name: **Physician ID#:**

HISTORY: Include significant positives and negatives from the HPI, past medical history, review of system(s), and social and family history.

CC: *Age, gender, presenting complaint*

HPI: *Site*
            Intensity/Quantity
            Quality
            Onset
            Radiation
            Alleviating and Aggravating factors
            Associated symptoms

PMH: *Previous episode, Dx, Tx*
            Allergies, general plus drugs
            Medications: Rx and non-Rx
            History of related illnesses/conditions, hospitalizations, surgery, trauma
            Review of systems

FH: *Same/similar complaint, related illnesses/conditions, other serious illnesses/conditions*

OB/GYN: *LMP, regular, duration, gravis, para, abortion/miscarriage, surgery, vaginal infections*

SxH: *Active, number of partners, M/F/B, condoms, STDs*

SH: *Habits (tobacco, alcohol, recreational drugs), work situation, home life*

PHYSICAL EXAMINATION: Indicate only pertinent positive and negative findings related to the patient's chief complaint.

VS: *WNL, except:*

General appearance: *Pt. supine in apparent distress, guarding RUQ*

Documentation of Body Systems/s Examined:
– Example of a normal abdominal system:
    Ø Surgical Scars or skin abnormalities on inspection
    Bowel sounds present + normoactive
    Abdomen tympanic to percussion in all 4 quadrants; no organomegaly
    Ø palpable masses, soft, nontender, nondistended to palpation
    Ø rebound or CVA tenderness
– Example of a normal CV system:
    Pulses 2+ BL
    PMI nondisplaced
    Ø palpable heaves, normal S1/S2, Ø S3.S4, regular rate + rhythm, Ø murmurs
    Ø rubs, gallops, JVD, or pedal edema

DIFFERENTIAL DIAGNOSIS
In order of likelihood (with 1 being most likely);
list 5 possible diagnoses:

1. *Most likely diagnosis*
2.
3.
4.
5. *Least likely diagnosis*

DIAGOSTIC WORKUP
List immediate plans (up to likely); list 5 possible diagnoses:

1   *Indicate specific first-line treatments in the order that they*
2. *would be performed in a lab setting. Use one line for all*
3. *related tasks.*
4.
5.

CLINICAL EXERCISE 4

Writing a Note

Five practice cases are presented below. Read the doorway (introductory) information, begin generating hypotheses, then read the history and physical examination. Write a note for those patient "encounters". When you are finished, compare your answers with those found in Appendix V.

Practice Case 1

Chart Information

Chief complaint: A 55-year-old man presents with lack of energy.

Vital signs: T: 36.6 C (98.0 F), BP: 154/96 mm Hg, HR: 48/min, RR: 12/min

History of Present Illness (HPI)

The patient made this appointment because he doesn't have enough energy and feels weak and tired. Even after a night of restful sleep, he feels fatigued early in the day. He's not entirely sure when this tiredness began, but it seems to have occurred little by little over the past 2 to 3 years. The patient has gained about 5 lb in the last year, but does not exercise as regularly as he used to. In the last year, his memory is not what it used to be either; he used to remember every one of his clients' names and now has difficulty with many of them. The patient's right hand feels funny, like it's asleep, especially when he wakes. He thinks it is probably his age, but he hasn't seen a doctor in about 2 years. He is a bank vice-president in charge of consumer loans.

Physical Examination

Mr. Ven is slightly overweight, and his voice sounds harsh. Vital signs are as noted. The skin on the front of each forearm is dry and scaly. Examination of the neck is normal. The apical impulse of the heart is not displaced, and no murmurs are audible. Abdominal examination discloses no abnormalities; the span of the liver in the right midclavicular line is 10 cm. Examination of the right hand reveals decreased pain sensation on the palm and the front of the thumb, index, and middle fingers.

Practice Case 1

HISTORY: Include significant positives and negatives from the history of present illness, past medical history, review of system(s), social history, and family history.

PHYSICAL EXAMINATION: Indicate only pertinent positive and negative findings related to the patient's chief complaint.

DIFFERENTIAL DIAGNOSIS

In order of likelihood (with 1 being most likely); list 5 possible diagnoses:

1.

2.

3.

4.

5.

DIAGNOSTIC WORKUP

List immediate plans (up to 5):

1.

2.

3.

4.

5.

Practice Case 2

Chart information

Chief complaint: A 42-year-old woman presents with chest pain.

Vital signs: T: 98.6 F (37 C), BP: 150/90 mm Hg, HR: 80/min, RR: 14/min

History

The pain began 10 hours ago. She describes it as a constant sharp pain across her chest; 5/10 in intensity. The pain does not radiate. There is no change in the pain with exercise, food, or deep inspiration. There is no associated shortness of breath or palpitations. She has never had this pain before and denies any recent injuries or hospitalizations. She relates no history of hypertension, heart disease, or diabetes. She is currently not taking any medication and has no allergies. Her menstrual period is regular, and the last one began 2 weeks ago. She has no history of any sexually transmitted diseases and has sex only with her husband of 15 years. There is no family history of similar chest pain or heart disease. The patient does not smoke or take illicit drugs. She drinks two glasses of wine per week.

Physical exam

Her cardiovascular exam revealed a normal S1/S2, with no murmurs and a regular rhythm. There was no jugular venous distension. Her lungs were clear to auscultation, with normal tactile fremitus, no dullness to percussion, and no clubbing or cyanosis. There was reproducible tenderness on sternum palpation. Her bowel sounds were normal, and her abdomen was nontender.

Practice Case 2

HISTORY: Include significant positives and negatives from the history of present illness, past medical history, review of system(s), social history, and family history.

PHYSICAL EXAMINATION: Indicate only pertinent positive and negative findings related to the patient's chief complaint.

DIFFERENTIAL DIAGNOSIS

In order of likelihood (with 1 being most likely); list 5 possible diagnoses:

1.

2.

3.

4.

5.

DIAGNOSTIC WORKUP

List immediate plans (up to 5):

1.

2.

3.

4.

5.

Practice Case 3

Chart information

Chief complaint: A 58-year-old man presents with severe pain in his left knee and left great toe.

Vital signs: T: 99.8 F, BP: 130/80 mm Hg, HR: 88/min, RR: 16/min

History

Five hours ago he was wakened by the onset of burning left knee and left great toe pain, which rapidly grew so bad that he could not stand the weight of the bedclothes on his leg. He related that the pain intensity was 9/10 and did not radiate. Over the next few hours, he noticed swelling of the knee and toe and that both felt hot to the touch. He then took two ibuprofen and noticed that much of the swelling and pain subsided (5/10). The patient denied a history of trauma, fever, arthritis, or migratory joint pains. On reflection, he did recall a milder, short episode of right great toe pain 4 years ago after his son's wedding, which improved with two doses of ibuprofen. Apart from mild obesity, there is no history of renal disease, hypertension, diabetes, or ischemic heart disease. The patient does not have any allergies. He is married, his wife being his only sexual partner. There is no history of sexually transmitted diseases. He sits mostly at work as an office supervisor. He has two healthy children. Although he does not drink on a regular basis, yesterday he had at least five beers and ate generous helpings of hamburgers, hot dogs, and barbecued ribs. He stopped smoking 10 years ago and takes no medication other than occasional acetaminophen or ibuprofen. His father died 10 years ago of lung cancer. His mother is alive and well. He has two brothers, both healthy. There is no family history of arthritis or joint problems.

Physical Exam

There are no lesions or scars on the left lower extremity. His left knee and great toe are tender to palpation with limited painful flexion/extension. There are no signs of warmth or edema on the left or right lower extremity. His sensation, muscle strength, and reflexes are intact and equal bilaterally. His pedal pulses are palpable and equal bilaterally.

Practice Case 3

HISTORY: Include significant positives and negatives from the history of present illness, past medical history, review of system(s), social history, and family history.

PHYSICAL EXAMINATION: Indicate only pertinent positive and negative findings related to the patient's chief complaint.

DIFFERENTIAL DIAGNOSIS

In order of likelihood (with 1 being most likely); list 5 possible diagnoses:

1.

2.

3.

4.

5.

DIAGNOSTIC WORKUP

List immediate plans (up to 5):

1.

2.

3.

4.

5.

Practice Case 4

Chart information

Chief complaint: A 58-year-old man presents with severe chest pain.

Vital signs: T: 98.6 F, BP: 128/80 mm Hg, HR: 110/min, RR: 22/min

History

One hour ago he developed sharp (7/10), substernal chest pain. There is no radiation of the pain. He is also somewhat short of breath, but is not diaphoretic or nauseated. The pain occurred while he was helping his son move his furniture into a new apartment. He tried resting, but is still in pain. There have been no prior episodes of pain, and he is generally healthy. He has a healthy diet and has not had any recent weight changes. He is a nonsmoker and does not drink alcohol. His father died at age 67 of "heart trouble." He has no allergies, and his only medications are vitamins. He is married, and his wife is his only sexual partner. He has no history of sexually transmitted diseases. He is a retired police officer and has three grown healthy children.

Physical exam

His chest is clear to auscultation bilaterally. The pain is not reproduced by palpation. Tactile fremitus is normal. There is no clubbing or cyanosis present. His heart demonstrated normal sounds, rate, and rhythm. There were no murmurs, gallops, or peripheral edema. JVD was not present. On abdominal exam, his liver was not enlarged. He had normal active bowel sounds, and his abdomen is tympanic to percussion in all four quadrants with no pain on abdominal palpation.

KAPLAN
medical

Practice Case 4

HISTORY: Include significant positives and negatives from the history of present illness, past medical history, review of system(s), social history, and family history.

PHYSICAL EXAMINATION: Indicate only pertinent positive and negative findings related to the patient's chief complaint.

DIFFERENTIAL DIAGNOSIS

In order of likelihood (with 1 being most likely); list 5 possible diagnoses:

1.

2.

3.

4.

5.

DIAGNOSTIC WORKUP

List immediate plans (up to 5):

1.

2.

3.

4.

5.

Practice Case 5

Chart information

Chief complaint: A 48-year-old woman presents with confusion, blurry vision, and shortness of breath.

Vital signs: T: 98.6 F, BP: 230/150 mm Hg, HR: 88/min, RR: 16/min

History

The patient presents with about 3 hours of dyspnea, blurry vision, and difficulty thinking. She has never had symptoms like this before. She is not sure why it started, and has noticed it has been getting slightly worse over the past hour or so. The symptoms came on when she was at her sedentary office job. She also complains of worsening headache, dizziness, and mild palpitations. She has not had fever, nausea, or vomiting. The patient has never had a myocardial infarction in the past, but she has high blood pressure for which she is on a thiazide diuretic. Otherwise, her past medical history is unremarkable. Her last period was 2 weeks ago, and she has been regular. She has had two normal pregnancies and has two healthy children in their twenties. She has maintained a good diet and has not had any weight or sleep changes. She does not have any allergies. She is not sexually active and has no history of sexually transmitted diseases. The patient is a nonsmoker, has about one glass of wine in a month, and does not use illegal drugs. Both parents are alive and healthy with no history of heart, lung, or blood pressure problems.

Physical exam

Her pupils were equal, round, and reactive to light and accommodation. Her extraocular movements are normal. Her visual field and examination of her external eye structures are normal. On ophthalmoscopic examination, the disc margins are sharp, with normal vasculature. Her heart demonstrates normal sounds, rate, and rhythm. There are no murmurs, gallops, or peripheral edema. JVD is not present. On abdominal exam, she has normal active bowel sounds. Her abdomen is tympanic to percussion in all four quadrants with no tenderness on palpation. Cranial nerve exam is normal. Reflexes, muscle strength, and sensation are normal in the upper and lower extremities.

Practice Case 5

HISTORY: Include significant positives and negatives from the history of present illness, past medical history, review of system(s), social history, and family history.

PHYSICAL EXAMINATION: Indicate only pertinent positive and negative findings related to the patient's chief complaint.

DIFFERENTIAL DIAGNOSIS	DIAGNOSTIC WORKUP
In order of likelihood (with 1 being most likely); list 5 possible diagnoses:	List immediate plans (up to 5):
1.	1.
2.	2.
3.	3.
4.	4.
5.	5.

Chapter Six: **Clinical Practice Cases**

The following 35 cases are designed to give you additional practice with Step 2 CS–style scenarios. They should be used after you have reviewed all of the material in this book.

As you review each case, use the margins as you would use scrap paper on the exam to write down any important findings. Begin to draw a mental picture of the patient and the differential diagnosis, and use the pages following the cases to predict what you think the history and physical exam checklist items would be. Then write a patient note, including the significant positives and negatives from the history and physical exam, and indicate your list of differential diagnoses and diagnostic workup plans.

Review your predictions and notes with the answers found in Appendix V.

PRACTICE CASE 1

Chart Information

Chief complaint: A 52-year-old man comes to the emergency department complaining of fatigue, cough, and chest pain.

Vital signs: T: 38.2 C (100.8 F), BP: 132/90 mm Hg, HR: 91/min, RR: 22/min, pulse oximetry: 92% on room air

History

The patient presents with a worsening cough that has developed slowly over the last 6 months. He is not sure exactly when or why the cough started, but feels it has been getting worse. He occasionally produces a small amount of rusty or blood-tinged sputum, although he describes his cough as mainly "dry and hacking." Over the last month or two, he has had episodes of chills and will often wake to find his sheets drenched in sweat. Additionally, over the last few days, he has suffered sharp, right-sided chest pain, which seems worse when he breathes deeply. The pain is rated a four on a one-to-ten scale and does not move to any other part of his body. His symptoms are mildly relieved with over-the-counter acetaminophen and cough suppressants. The patient denies ever having these symptoms in the past, although he does note that he has had recurrent episodes of "pneumonia" over the last year or two. He denies any episodes of orthopnea, acute shortness of breath, nausea, or diaphoresis. The patient has had a 20-lb weight loss over the last four months and states that he just "doesn't feel hungry." Aside from these episodes of self-diagnosed pneumonia, he reports having no major illnesses, hospitalizations, or past operations, although he did once have "the clap" three years ago, diagnosed after suffering from a painful penile discharge. He is not allergic to any medications and does not usually take any, prescription or otherwise. The patient has not traveled recently and cannot think of any recent sick contacts, although he states that he was recently released from prison, where his long-term cellmate had a "nasty cough." The patient admits to a history of heroin use and having sex with men, stating that he "did what I had to do" while in prison. Additionally, he smoked one to two packs of cigarettes per day for the last 35 years, but denies drinking alcohol. Both of his parents are alive, and he knows of no illnesses in his family.

Physical Examination

Head and neck exam shows a normal oropharynx with no oral ulcers or evidence of thrush. Lymph node exam reveals no obvious cervical, supraclavicular, or axillary lymphadenopathy. His chest is clear to auscultation and percussion, and tactile fremitus is within normal limits. The patient grimaces with deep inspiration and coughs on expiration. His chest wall is not tender, and there is no clubbing or cyanosis present. His heart demonstrates normal sounds, rate, and rhythm, without any murmurs, rubs, gallops, or peripheral edema. Jugular venous pressure is within normal limits. Abdominal exam fails to reveal any hepatosplenomegaly. He has normal, active bowel sounds, and his abdomen is tympanic to percussion in all four quadrants, with no pain or tenderness present on palpation. Examination of his skin reveals two, non-tender, reddish-purple, half-inch round spots on the left shin, as well as a poorly done tattoo on his left chest.

Practice Case 1

Standardized Patient History-Taking Checklist

1.

2.

3.

4.

5.

6.

7.

8.

9.

10.

11.

12.

13.

14.

Standardized Patient Physical Examination Checklist

1.

2.

3.

4.

5.

6.

7.

8.

9.

10.

11.

12.

KAPLAN
medical

HISTORY: Include significant positives and negatives from the history of present illness, past medical history, review of system(s), social history, and family history.

PHYSICAL EXAMINATION: Indicate only pertinent positive and negative findings related to the patient's chief complaint.

DIFFERENTIAL DIAGNOSIS

In order of likelihood (with 1 being most likely); list 5 possible diagnoses:

1.

2.

3.

4.

5.

DIAGNOSTIC WORKUP

List immediate plans (up to 5):

1.

2.

3.

4.

5.

PRACTICE CASE 2

Chart Information

Chief complaint: A 31-year-old man comes to the clinic with chest and stomach pain.

Vital signs: T: 98.6 F (37 C), BP: 130/85 mm Hg, HR: 108/min, RR: 16/min

History

For approximately a year, this patient has suffered a burning, epigastric pain (4/10). The pain is located in the center of his stomach, occasionally in his lower chest, and seems to spread through to his back. The pain occasionally wakes the patient at night, although it does not seem to be associated with any constitutional symptoms. He has not suffered any night sweats, fevers, chills, or significant weight loss, nor has he had any recent diaphoresis, shortness of breath, nausea, or vomiting. He does, however, occasionally suffer from a burning sensation and foul taste in his throat. Recently, the pain has become more frequent and more painful, and the patient has had some episodes of dark stools, although he has never noticed any blood in his stool. Eating seems to help with the pain, as do over-the-counter antacids. The pain does not appear to be related to exertion. Aside from over-the-counter antacids, the patient takes no medications, prescriptions, or otherwise, and specifically denies taking any nonsteroidal anti-inflammatory medications. He is single and works as an investment banker. He has an erratic diet, eating when he can (usually fast food), and admits to a 20-pack-year history of tobacco and a near-daily consumption of one to two gin and tonics to help him relax from the stresses of work. He denies using illicit drugs. Occasionally, the alcohol may worsen his symptoms. Aside from his current symptoms, which he has not suffered before this year, he has no other medical problems and is unaware of any medical problems in his family. He specifically denies any history of diabetes, heart disease, or elevated lipid levels in himself or close family members.

Physical Examination

His chest is clear to auscultation bilaterally, and tactile fremitus is within normal limits. His cardiac exam demonstrates normal sounds, rate, and rhythm, without any murmurs, rubs, or peripheral edema. His jugular venous pressure is about 7 cm H_2O. On abdominal exam, his liver and spleen are not enlarged. He has normal active bowel sounds, and his abdomen is tympanic to percussion in all four quadrants. He is mildly tender to palpation in the midepigastric area, but displays no rebound tenderness or guarding. He has a negative Murphy sign. Of note, the patient states he normally is much darker skinned than he is currently.

Practice Case 2

Standardized Patient History-Taking Checklist

1.

2.

3.

4.

5.

6.

7.

8.

9.

10.

11.

12.

13.

14.

15.

Standardized Patient Physical Examination Checklist

1.

2.

3.

4.

5.

6.

7.

8.

9.

HISTORY: Include significant positives and negatives from the history of present illness, past medical history, review of system(s), social history, and family history.

PHYSICAL EXAMINATION: Indicate only pertinent positive and negative findings related to the patient's chief complaint.

DIFFERENTIAL DIAGNOSIS

In order of likelihood (with 1 being most likely); list 5 possible diagnoses:

1.

2.

3.

4.

5.

DIAGNOSTIC WORKUP

List immediate plans (up to 5):

1.

2.

3.

4.

5.

PRACTICE CASE 3

Chart Information

Chief complaint: A 63-year-old woman has back pain and fever.

Vital signs: T: 38.3 C (101.0 F), BP: 129/85 mm Hg, HR: 108/min, RR: 16/min

History

The patient's problems started about 3 days ago, when she felt nauseated and fatigued. She tried to rest, which helped her symptoms minimally, but had to get up frequently to urinate. Assuming she had the flu, she stayed in bed and drank fluids, waiting for her illness to pass. However, about a day after her symptoms began, she began to have chills and fevers, as well as pain over her right lower back. The pain is dull, poorly localized, and mainly over the right lumbar area. Additionally, she has had some mild pain over the lower part of her abdomen. The pain is fairly constant, does not move to any other location, and is rated 4/10 in severity. In addition to chills, fevers, fatigue, and episodic nausea, she reports muscle and joint pains and headaches. Some over-the-counter acetaminophen has helped her symptoms, but otherwise, not much seems to make them better or worse. Prior to this event, she has been relatively healthy, although she suffers from noninsulin-dependent diabetes mellitus. In addition to diabetes, which is usually well controlled, she has a history of recurrent urinary tract infections, hypertension, kidney stones, and a diabetic foot ulcer. Her blood pressure normally has a "top" number in the 140s. She currently takes only metformin and lisinopril and has no known drug allergies. Since feeling ill, she has not taken either medication. She does report having somewhat similar symptoms with a urinary tract infection one year ago, but states this is much worse. Currently, she is suffering from some mild pain with urination and occasional urinary incontinence, but denies any blood or changes in the appearance of her urine. Although she is nauseated, she is able to tolerate an oral diet without vomiting. She has not had any changes in her weight or appetite, although she had recently reduced her fluid intake as part of a crash diet. Her family history includes a mother with diabetes. Her last menstrual period was ten years ago, and she has not had any vaginal discharge. She does not drink, smoke, or use illicit drugs.

Physical Examination

The patient appears flushed, in mild discomfort, and appears anxious. Her skin feels mildly warm to touch. Her chest is clear to auscultation bilaterally, and tactile fremitus is normal. Cardiac exam reveals normal heart sounds, rate, and rhythm. There are no murmurs, rubs, or gallops. Jugular venous pressure is less than 5 cm. Her extremities show no evidence of cyanosis, clubbing, or edema. On abdominal exam, there is no evidence of hepatosplenomegaly by percussion, and the abdomen is tympanic in all four quadrants. She has normal active bowel sounds, but is mildly tender to palpation in the lower aspect of her abdomen. She has significant right costovertebral angle tenderness. There are no surgical scars or palpable masses present. She does not display guarding or rebound tenderness, and has a negative Murphy sign. At the end of the exam, she stands up, but has to lean against the exam table because she feels "woozy".

Practice Case 3

Standardized Patient History-Taking Checklist

1.

2.

3.

4.

5.

6.

7.

8.

9.

10.

11.

12.

13.

14.

15.

16.

Standardized Patient Physical Examination Checklist

1.

2.

3.

4.

5.

6.

7.

8.

9.

10.

HISTORY: Include significant positives and negatives from the history of present illness, past medical history, review of system(s), social history, and family history.

PHYSICAL EXAMINATION: Indicate only pertinent positive and negative findings related to the patient's chief complaint.

DIFFERENTIAL DIAGNOSIS

In order of likelihood (with 1 being most likely); list 5 possible diagnoses:

1.

2.

3.

4.

5.

DIAGNOSTIC WORKUP

List immediate plans (up to 5):

1.

2.

3.

4.

5.

PRACTICE CASE 4

Chart Information

Chief complaint: A 72-year-old woman comes to the emergency department with rectal bleeding.

Vital signs: T: 36.7 C (98.0 F), BP: 108/55 mm Hg, HR: 109/min, RR: 16/min

History

This patient noticed bright red blood in the toilet bowl earlier in the afternoon. The blood appeared to fill the entire bowl, although she is not exactly sure how much she bled. Since then, she has had three additional bloody bowel movements, with the last bowel movement occurring 1 hour ago. The blood is mixed in with the stool and is also present on the toilet paper. There is no pain or cramping associated with her bowel movements, although she does now admit to feeling weak and dizzy, but she has not had any palpitations or altered mental status. Prior to this afternoon, she has been in her usual state of health and denies any fevers, chills, nausea, vomiting, melena, dysuria, or weight loss. There have been no changes in her bowel habits or stools, and she cannot think of a precipitating event. She is not allergic to any medications, denies any use of nonsteroidal anti-inflammatories, and takes only hydrochlorothiazide (which she did not take this morning), a multivitamin, and occasional acetaminophen. She has had no changes in her diet, has not traveled anywhere, and denies any sick contacts. She does not drink, smoke, or use any illicit substances. The patient has never bled before and does not believe anyone in her family has had a similar problem or has suffered from gastrointestinal illness or cancer. Her past medical illnesses include hypertension (untreated systolic pressures in the 160s), osteoporosis, diverticulitis, and a cholecystectomy in her forties. She has never had any colon cancer screening.

Physical Examination

The patient is sitting comfortably on the exam table. Her chest is clear to auscultation bilaterally. Cardiovascular exam demonstrates normal sounds, rate and rhythm, without any murmurs, rubs, or gallops. Jugular veins appear flat. On abdominal exam, percussion and palpation do not reveal an enlarged liver or spleen. She has normal active bowel sounds, and the abdomen is tympanic to percussion in all four quadrants. There is no tenderness to palpation in any quadrant, and no masses are palpable. Her skin appears normal, without evidence of a rash, although there is an old, well-healed surgical scar in the right upper quadrant.

Practice Case 4

Standardized Patient History-Taking Checklist

1.

2.

3.

4.

5.

6.

7.

8.

9.

10.

11.

12.

13.

14.

15.

Standardized Patient Physical Examination Checklist

1.

2.

3.

4.

5.

6.

7.

8.

9.

HISTORY: Include significant positives and negatives from the history of present illness, past medical history, review of system(s), social history, and family history.

PHYSICAL EXAMINATION: Indicate only pertinent positive and negative findings related to the patient's chief complaint.

DIFFERENTIAL DIAGNOSIS

In order of likelihood (with 1 being most likely); list 5 possible diagnoses:

1.

2.

3.

4.

5.

DIAGNOSTIC WORKUP

List immediate plans (up to 5):

1.

2.

3.

4.

5.

PRACTICE CASE 5

Chart Information

Chief complaint: A 48-year-old woman comes in with chest pain.

Vital signs: T: 38.0 C (100.4 F), BP: 128/58 mm Hg, HR: 109/min, RR: 26/min

History

Four hours ago, while collecting her luggage after a trip to Japan, she developed sharp (6/10) substernal chest pain. There is no movement of the pain, and she is not diaphoretic or nauseated, but has developed significant difficulty catching her breath. She originally thought her chest pain was due to lifting her heavy luggage. However, her symptoms have not improved with rest or over-the-counter acetaminophen. Breathing or sudden movement seems to make the pain worse. Prior to this, she has never had chest pain and has generally been healthy. Specifically, she has not had any recent fevers, chills, cough, dysuria, weight or appetite changes, difficulty sleeping, or sick contacts. The patient has not suffered any episodes of shortness of breath, pain, lower extremity swelling, or orthopnea. She suffers from borderline hypertension (which is diet controlled), had an appendectomy as a child, and has only been hospitalized for the birth of her two children. There is no history of heart disease, diabetes, or elevated cholesterol in her or family members. She takes oral contraceptive pills to help regulate her menstrual cycles, acetaminophen, and a multivitamin, and has no known drug allergies. She admits to smoking about half a pack of cigarettes since age 20, although she is currently trying to quit. The patient drinks only rarely at social events and does not use any illicit substances. She is married, works as a corporate lawyer, and her husband is her only sexual partner.

Physical Examination

The patient appears anxious and uncomfortable. She appears to be breathing at a rate of approximately 25 to 30 breaths/min. She is not using any accessory muscles of respiration, and her chest wall appears symmetrical. Her chest is clear to auscultation bilaterally, but she has difficulty complying with the exam, as deep breaths are extremely painful. The pain is not reproduced by palpation and is not affected by positioning. Tactile fremitus is normal. There is no cyanosis, clubbing, or edema present. Her heart demonstrates normal sounds, rate, and rhythm. There were no murmurs, rubs, or gallops present. The point of maximal impulse is not displaced. Pulses are normal and equal in strength bilaterally. The top of her jugular venous fluid column appears at approximately 2 cm above her sternoclavicular notch. On abdominal exam, the liver is not enlarged. She has normal active bowel sounds, and the abdomen is tympanic to percussion in all four quadrants with no pain on palpation. A small, well-healed surgical scar is present in her right-lower quadrant. There are no lower extremity varicosities, tenderness, or palpable cords.

Practice Case 5

Standardized Patient History-Taking Checklist

1.

2.

3.

4.

5.

6.

7.

8.

9.

10.

11.

12.

13.

14.

15.

16.

17.

Standardized Patient Physical Examination Checklist

1.

2.

3.

4.

5.

6.

7.

8.

9.

10.

11.

HISTORY: Include significant positives and negatives from the history of present illness, past medical history, review of system(s), social history, and family history.

PHYSICAL EXAMINATION: Indicate only pertinent positive and negative findings related to the patient's chief complaint.

DIFFERENTIAL DIAGNOSIS

In order of likelihood (with 1 being most likely); list 5 possible diagnoses:

1.

2.

3.

4.

5.

DIAGNOSTIC WORKUP

List immediate plans (up to 5):

1.

2.

3.

4.

5.

PRACTICE CASE 6

Chart Information

Chief complaint:	A 29-year-old man comes to the emergency department complaining of a severe headache.
Vital signs:	T: 37.8 C (100 F), BP: 169/108 mm Hg, HR: 48/min, RR: 12/min

History

The pain began about 4 hours ago, waking him from sleep. The pain is described as relentless, lancinating, and diffuse, with a severity of 10/10. It is difficult to localize, but seems to shoot down his neck and back if he coughs or quickly moves his head. The patient has never had a headache this severe, although he did have a moderately painful (6/10) headache one day prior to his current symptoms. He reports feeling nauseated, although he has not vomited. He has not had a loss of consciousness, denies a history of trauma, and has not had any seizure-like activity. Prior to this event, the patient has not suffered from any fevers, chills, confusion, changes in vision, or recent upper respiratory infections and is generally in good health. Over-the-counter medications have not helped control the pain. He takes no regular medications (specifically, no cough remedies or appetite suppressants) or herbal supplements and has no known drug allergies. The patient suffers from no medical illnesses, although he has an uncle on dialysis for complications of polycystic kidney disease. His family history is otherwise unremarkable; there is no history of stroke, vascular disease, or heart disease. He admits to drinking alcohol nearly daily, has smoked one to two packs of cigarettes a day for the past ten years, and occasionally uses intranasal cocaine, although no intravenous drugs. He last used cocaine the prior evening. He is monogamous with his wife, has no other sexual partners, and works as a bartender.

Physical Examination

The patient is in moderate pain and appears confused, having difficulty remembering the date and focusing on the examination. His head appears normal, without any evidence of trauma. He is able to track the movements of your finger with his eyes, but shies away from the ophthalmoscope, stating that the light is painful. With great effort, a funduscopic exam is performed, which does not reveal any lesions or optic disc blurring. The rest of his cranial nerves are intact. Motor strength is normal in all muscle groups, as is sensation to sharp, dull, and proprioceptive stimuli. His deep tendon reflexes are normal. The patient is able to touch his nose and then touch your finger, and, when standing upright with arms extended, does not lose his balance when he closes his eyes. His toes are downgoing when the dorsolateral aspect of the foot is rubbed with the reflex hammer. The patient reports tenderness with flexion of the neck and pain with extension of the leg when the thigh is flexed. Auscultation of the lungs reveals clear lung fields. Cardiac exam reveals normal heart sounds, with no murmurs, rubs, or gallops. Peripheral pulses are normal. Examination of the extremities reveals no clubbing, cyanosis, edema, or stigmata of endocarditis. The patient's abdomen is soft, nontender, and nondistended, and no masses are felt.

Practice Case 6

Standardized Patient History-Taking Checklist

1.

2.

3.

4.

5.

6.

7.

8.

9.

10.

11.

12.

13.

14.

15.

Standardized Patient Physical Examination Checklist

1.

2.

3.

4.

5.

6.

7.

8.

9.

10.

11.

12.

13.

14.

15.

HISTORY: Include significant positives and negatives from the history of present illness, past medical history, review of system(s), social history, and family history.

PHYSICAL EXAMINATION: Indicate only pertinent positive and negative findings related to the patient's chief complaint.

DIFFERENTIAL DIAGNOSIS

In order of likelihood (with 1 being most likely); list 5 possible diagnoses:

1.

2.

3.

4.

5.

DIAGNOSTIC WORKUP

List immediate plans (up to 5):

1.

2.

3.

4.

5.

PRACTICE CASE 7

Chart Information

Chief complaint: A 31-year-old woman comes to the emergency department complaining of severe abdominal pain.

Vital signs: T: 38.3 C (101.0 F), BP: 102/60 mm Hg, HR: 109/min, RR: 27/min

History

The pain began suddenly 5 hours ago. It is severe (10/10), described as a constant, aching pain and is located mainly in the upper part of the patient's abdomen. The pain spreads in a band-like pattern to the back. The patient tried to treat the pain by drinking a fifth of vodka and taking some aspirin, neither of which helped. The only thing that seems to help the pain is leaning forward; the patient definitely thinks the pain is worse when she lies down. She denies having any recent fever, chills, diarrhea, cough, chest pain, or dark stools, and has not been around any sick people. She does have a mild sensation of being short of breath. Additionally, shortly after consuming the vodka, she vomited three times, although she is not sure if there was any blood present. The patient has had one episode of similar pain 2 years ago. Unfortunately, she is unable to provide much information, as she was in the intensive care unit and does not know what her diagnosis was. She takes no medications and has no drug allergies. Her past medical history includes alcoholism, gallstones, and recurrent urinary tract infections, although she has not had any recent urinary tract infection symptoms. Her mother suffers from diabetes, and her father has high blood pressure, but both are alive and well. She denies any history of sexually transmitted diseases, is monogamous and uses condoms, and has no children. Her menstrual periods have been normal, with the last one two weeks ago. Currently, she is unemployed and admits to drinking regularly to deal with the frustration. Her last drink was earlier in the day. She does not smoke or use any illicit substances.

Physical Examination

The patient appears anxious, is unable to sit still, and appears moderately uncomfortable. Her chest is clear to auscultation bilaterally. Her heart demonstrates normal sounds, rate, and rhythm, without any murmurs, rubs, or gallops. Jugular venous pressure appears normal. On abdominal exam, the patient is tender to palpation diffusely, but worse in the midepigastrium and right upper quadrants. Voluntary guarding is present, although there is no rebound tenderness. Bowel sounds are normal, and the abdomen is tympanic to percussion in all four quadrants. There is no discoloration on the abdomen or flanks, and no costovertebral angle tenderness is present. Although she has significant right upper quadrant tenderness, a Murphy sign is not present. Rovsing, obturator, and iliopsoas signs are also not present. Extremities show no evidence of cyanosis, clubbing, or edema.

Practice Case 7

Standardized Patient History-Taking Checklist

1.

2.

3.

4.

5.

6.

7.

8.

9.

10.

11.

12.

13.

14.

15.

16.

17.

Standardized Patient Physical Examination Checklist

1.

2.

3.

4.

5.

6.

7.

8.

9.

10.

11.

HISTORY: Include significant positives and negatives from the history of present illness, past medical history, review of system(s), social history, and family history.

PHYSICAL EXAMINATION: Indicate only pertinent positive and negative findings related to the patient's chief complaint.

DIFFERENTIAL DIAGNOSIS

In order of likelihood (with 1 being most likely); list 5 possible diagnoses:

1.

2.

3.

4.

5.

DIAGNOSTIC WORKUP

List immediate plans (up to 5):

1.

2.

3.

4.

5.

PRACTICE CASE 8

Chart Information

Chief complaint: A 19-year-old woman presents with abdominal pain.

Vital signs: T: 37.1 C (98.8 F), BP: 118/82 mm Hg, HR: 82/min, RR: 16/min

History

The pain began about one day ago. It is located in the middle, lower part of her abdomen and seems to be worse with urination. On a pain scale of one to ten, the patient rates the pain a four that does not move to any other location. She denies seeing any blood in her urine, but notes that it has appeared cloudy. Practically every half hour to an hour, she needs to urinate. Further, when the urge to urinate occurs, she can barely make it to a bathroom in time. To help with the pain, she has taken acetaminophen and, on the advice of friends, large amounts of cranberry juice, neither of which have provided much relief. She has had no back pain, fever, chills, vaginal discharge, or gastrointestinal complaints and has generally been in good health, never having had a major illness or hospitalization. This has never happened before. She has no other medical problems and takes no medications, prescription or otherwise, and has no known drug allergies. Her mother, father, and two sisters are alive and well; however, her mother has hypertension. The patient occasionally drinks at parties, but does not smoke or use drugs. She is sexually active with her boyfriend, who is her only sexual partner. Indeed, she states that she just recently had sex for the first time. They do not use condoms, and she reports never having had a sexually transmitted disease in the past. Her last menstrual period was 2 weeks ago and was normal.

Physical Examination

The patient appears comfortable. Her lungs are clear to auscultation bilaterally. Her cardiovascular exam reveals normal heart sounds, with no murmurs, rubs, or gallops. On abdominal exam, percussion and palpation do not reveal an enlarged liver or spleen. She has normal active bowel sounds, and the abdomen is tympanic to percussion in all four quadrants. There is mild tenderness on palpation of the lower abdomen. No costovertebral angle tenderness is present. Her skin shows no discoloration, rash, or lesions. The patient's extremities reveal no evidence of cyanosis, clubbing, or edema.

Practice Case 8

Standardized Patient History-Taking Checklist

1.

2.

3.

4.

5.

6.

7.

8.

9.

10.

11.

12.

13.

14.

15.

16.

17.

18.

Standardized Patient Physical Examination Checklist

1.

2.

3.

4.

5.

6.

7.

8.

9.

HISTORY: Include significant positives and negatives from the history of present illness, past medical history, review of system(s), social history, and family history.

PHYSICAL EXAMINATION: Indicate only pertinent positive and negative findings related to the patient's chief complaint.

DIFFERENTIAL DIAGNOSIS

In order of likelihood (with 1 being most likely); list 5 possible diagnoses:

1.

2.

3.

4.

5.

DIAGNOSTIC WORKUP

List immediate plans (up to 5):

1.

2.

3.

4.

5.

KAPLAN
medical

PRACTICE CASE 9

Chart Information

Chief complaint: A 65-year-old-man comes the clinic complaining of difficulty sleeping because of the need to urinate.

Vital signs: T: 37.0 C (98.6 F), BP: 130/85 mm Hg, HR: 82/min, RR: 16/min

History

Over the last 2 years, the patient has had difficulty sleeping. He reports waking at least three to four times a night to urinate. Despite these frequent attempts at urination, he often feels that he cannot "get it all out." During the daytime, he also has to frequently urinate, although it is sometimes difficult to initiate urination. When he does urinate, the stream is weak, and there is often posturination dribbling. He denies any pain or blood with urination, has not had any changes in appetite or weight, and denies any body or back pain. He has not had any fevers, chills, penile discharge, or nausea. In general, he reports feeling otherwise healthy. He has tried to relieve his symptoms by minimizing the amount of water he drinks at night, but this has not provided any relief. Nothing he can think of exacerbates his condition. The symptoms, which began insidiously, now seem to be getting worse. Prior to these last 2 years, he has not had any urinary problems. The patient is not allergic to any medications and takes hydrochlorothiazide and amitriptyline for high blood pressure and depression, respectively. He states that both of these problems are well controlled. Additionally, the patient was diagnosed with diabetes mellitus 1 year ago. Currently, he controls his blood sugar with diet and exercise. There are no illnesses that run in his family. He is not currently sexually active, having "lost the ability" a few years back. He was once sexually active, when in the Navy, and had two episodes of a penile discharge treated "with a shot in butt." He does not drink or use tobacco and has never used illicit drugs.

Physical Examination

The patient is sitting comfortably on the exam table. His chest is clear to auscultation bilaterally. Cardiovascular exam demonstrates normal sounds, rate, and rhythm, without any murmurs, rubs, or gallops. The top of the jugular venous column appears at about 2 cm above the sternal notch. On abdominal exam, percussion and palpation do not reveal an enlarged liver or spleen. He has normal active bowel sounds, and the abdomen is tympanic to percussion in all four quadrants. There is no tenderness to palpation in any quadrant, and no masses are palpable. There is no costovertebral angle tenderness. Sensation is intact to sharp, dull, and proprioception, and lower extremity muscle strength is normal. Deep tendon reflexes in the lower extremities are normal. When the feet are stroked on the lateral plantar edge, the patient curls his toes and withdraws his feet.

Practice Case 9

Standardized Patient History-Taking Checklist

1.

2.

3.

4.

5.

6.

7.

8.

9.

10.

11.

12.

13.

14.

15.

Standardized Patient Physical Examination Checklist

1.

2.

3.

4.

5.

6.

7.

8.

9.

10.

11.

12.

KAPLAN medical

HISTORY: Include significant positives and negatives from the history of present illness, past medical history, review of system(s), social history, and family history.

PHYSICAL EXAMINATION: Indicate only pertinent positive and negative findings related to the patient's chief complaint.

DIFFERENTIAL DIAGNOSIS

In order of likelihood (with 1 being most likely); list 5 possible diagnoses:

1.

2.

3.

4.

5.

DIAGNOSTIC WORKUP

List immediate plans (up to 5):

1.

2.

3.

4.

5.

PRACTICE CASE 10

Chart Information

Chief complaint: A 66-year-old man comes to the emergency department complaining
                          of weakness and a facial droop.

Vital signs: T: 37.0 C (98.6 F), BP: 151/90 mm Hg, HR: 77/min, RR: 14/min

History

About half an hour ago, the patient suffered a 20-min episode of slurred speech, right facial
droop and numbness, and weakness in his right arm. According to the patient's friend, who was
present for the episode, the patient was confused and distant immediately prior to and during
the attack. Further, when he did try to respond to questions, he would slur his speech. The
patient is now well and states his symptoms have completely resolved. He denies any recent
fevers, chills, weakness, seizure activity, and any episodes of altered mental status, recent falls,
vertigo, or headaches. He did not become incontinent of bowel or bladder or lose consciousness. The patient does admit to having two previous episodes of sudden, transient, right-sided
blindness, but denies any chest pain, palpitations, or shortness of breath. He did once have
weakness like this, about a week ago. Because it resolved in less than 5 minutes, he decided not
to seek medical help. He is not allergic to any medications and takes lisinopril, a daily baby
aspirin, metformin, and atorvastatin. The patient has a history of hypertension, diabetes, and
hyperlipidemia. There is no history of heart disease or stroke in the family, although the patient
states he was adopted. The patient does not drink and has never used street drugs, but admits
to smoking a pack a day since age 16.

Physical Examination

The patient is resting comfortably on the exam table. He is alert and oriented to person, place,
and date and is able to concentrate and complete the exam. He is able to track the movements
of your finger with his eyes and has a normal funduscopic exam. The rest of his cranial nerves
are intact. Motor strength is normal in all muscle groups, as is sensation to sharp, dull, and
vibratory stimuli. His deep tendon reflexes are normal. The patient is able to touch his nose and
then touch your finger and, when standing upright with arms extended, does not lose his balance when he closes his eyes. His toes are downgoing when the dorsolateral aspect of the foot is
rubbed with the reflex hammer. The patient walks normally without any unsteadiness.
Auscultation of the chest reveals clear lung fields. Cardiac exam reveals normal heart sounds,
with no murmurs, rubs, or gallops. The patient has a normal carotid upstroke, and the point of
maximal impulse is normal in size and location. Peripheral pulses are normal, and no carotid
bruits are heard. Examination of the extremities reveals no clubbing, cyanosis, edema, or signs
or stigmata of endocarditis. The patient's abdomen is soft, nontender, and nondistended, and
no masses are felt.

Practice Case 10

Standardized Patient History-Taking Checklist

1.

2.

3.

4.

5.

6.

7.

8.

9.

10.

11.

12.

13.

14.

15.

16.

Standardized Patient Physical Examination Checklist

1.

2.

3.

4.

5.

6.

7.

8.

9.

10.

11.

12.

13.

14.

15.

16.

HISTORY: Include significant positives and negatives from the history of present illness, past medical history, review of system(s), social history, and family history.

PHYSICAL EXAMINATION: Indicate only pertinent positive and negative findings related to the patient's chief complaint.

DIFFERENTIAL DIAGNOSIS

In order of likelihood (with 1 being most likely); list 5 possible diagnoses:

1.

2.

3.

4.

5.

DIAGNOSTIC WORKUP

List immediate plans (up to 5):

1.

2.

3.

4.

5.

PRACTICE CASE 11

Chart Information

Chief complaint: A 40-year-old man comes to the emergency department complaining of foot pain that woke him from sleep.

Vital signs: T: 38.0 C (100.5 F), BP: 158/90 mm Hg, HR: 88/min, RR: 14/min

History

Yesterday morning, the patient woke up and felt a throbbing pain in his left toe. At first, he ignored the pain. He was quite hungover from drinking with friends the night before and figured the pain would resolve spontaneously. However, over the course of the day, the pain became worse. It started at a 4/10 intensity and eventually peaked to an 8/10. The pain was located mainly in his great toe, although at times his entire foot ached, particularly when walking. There was no pain in any other joint, and aside from his toe pain, and perhaps a fever (he felt warm, but did not check his temperature), the patient reports feeling "okay." The patient has trouble thinking of a precipitating cause, but thinks he may have stubbed his toe while dancing on the bar of an after-hours club. The toe improved with high doses of indomethacin, which the patient was given the last time this happened. Apparently, he has had trouble like this twice in the past, once severe enough to prompt an emergency room visit. Further, a couple of weeks ago, he had severe pain in his right knee, as well as some overlying skin discoloration. He is not allergic to any medications and takes hydrochlorothiazide for high blood pressure. He denies any urinary or gastrointestinal changes. The patient works as a pharmaceutical representative and often consumes meals consisting of steak, shellfish, and liberal amounts of alcohol while entertaining important clients. Family history is unremarkable. The patient consumes a moderate amount of alcohol, drinking a glass or two of wine on most days, and getting drunk once a week, usually on the weekends. He does not feel concerned, angry, or guilty about his drinking and does not drink in the morning. And although he drinks regularly, he does not smoke and has never used any illicit drugs. He reports having four female sexual partners in the last month, and he usually uses condoms. He has never had any sexually transmitted diseases.

Physical Examination

The patient is sitting comfortably on the examination table. His chest is clear to auscultation bilaterally. Cardiovascular exam demonstrates normal sounds, rate, and rhythm, without any murmurs, rubs, or gallops. Jugular veins appear normal. On abdominal exam, he has normal active bowel sounds, and the abdomen is tympanic to percussion in all four quadrants. There is no tenderness to palpation in any quadrant, and no masses are palpable. His left big toe is cool to touch and does not feel deformed, although the patient grimaces with active and passive movement of the digit. The toe does not appear or feel to have a bony deformity or fracture. There is no effusion. The rest of the patient's joints do not appear inflamed, and no bony deformities or nodules are palpable. He has no rash or skin lesions.

Practice Case 11

Standardized Patient History-Taking Checklist

1.
2.
3.
4.
5.
6.
7.
8.
9.
10.
11.
12.
13.
14.
15.
16.
17.
18.
19.

Standardized Patient Physical Examination Checklist

1.
2.
3.
4.
5.
6.
7.
8.
9.
10.
11.
12.

HISTORY: Include significant positives and negatives from the history of present illness, past medical history, review of system(s), social history, and family history.

PHYSICAL EXAMINATION: Indicate only pertinent positive and negative findings related to the patient's chief complaint.

DIFFERENTIAL DIAGNOSIS	DIAGNOSTIC WORKUP
In order of likelihood (with 1 being most likely); list 5 possible diagnoses:	List immediate plans (up to 5):
1.	1.
2.	2.
3.	3.
4.	4.
5.	5.

PRACTICE CASE 12

Chart Information

Chief complaint: A 26-year-old Caucasian man has abdominal pain, vomiting, and increased urination.

Vital signs: T: 37.0 C (98.6 F), BP: 108/72 mm Hg, HR: 77/min, RR: 26/min

History

Over the last 24 hours, the patient has had increasing diffuse, dull, abdominal pain, and lethargy. The pain is rated a 4 out of 10. When he woke this morning, he had one episode of nonbloody vomiting. He has not had any fevers, chills, cough, diarrhea, or painful urination but reports that he has been going to the bathroom frequently. Indeed, over the past few weeks to a month, he has been thirsty all the time, has had frequent urination, and has lost 10 pounds, despite a "monster appetite." He also has suffered some visual changes. Every now and then, his vision will suddenly become blurry. The patient cannot think of any sick contacts and has not had any changes in his diet. Nothing seems to make these symptoms better or worse. These sorts of symptoms have never occurred before, and he has generally been quite healthy. He takes no medications, has no drug allergies, and has never spent a day in the hospital. The patient is a graduate student working in an endocrinology lab. Family members inspired his career; both of his parents and his maternal aunt have diabetes mellitus, although he is not sure which type. He does not smoke or drink alcohol, has never used drugs, is monogamous with one partner (a girlfriend), and uses condoms regularly.

Physical Examination

The patient is resting on the examination table and appears mildly uncomfortable. He is able to track the movements of your finger with his eyes, has a normal papillary response, and has no abnormalities on funduscopic exam. The rest of his cranial nerves are intact. Motor strength is normal in all muscle groups, as is sensation to sharp, dull, and vibratory stimuli. His deep tendon reflexes are normal. Auscultation of the chest reveals clear lung fields, and tactile fremitus is within normal limits. The patient is breathing deeply at a rate of 25 to 30/min, and his breath does not smell fruity. Cardiac exam reveals normal heart sounds, with no murmurs, rubs, or gallops. Examination of the extremities reveals no clubbing, cyanosis, or edema. Specifically, there are no lesions on the patient's feet. He has normal active bowel sounds, and the abdomen is tympanic to percussion in all four quadrants. There is no tenderness to palpation in any quadrant, and no masses are palpable. No rash or skin lesions are present. At the end of the exam, the patient states he feels nauseous and dizzy.

Practice Case 12

Standardized Patient History-Taking Checklist

1.

2.

3.

4.

5.

6.

7.

8.

9.

10.

11.

12.

13.

14.

15.

16.

17.

Standardized Patient Physical Examination Checklist

1.

2.

3.

4.

5.

6.

7.

8.

9.

10.

11.

KAPLAN
medical

HISTORY: Include significant positives and negatives from the history of present illness, past medical history, review of system(s), social history, and family history.

PHYSICAL EXAMINATION: Indicate only pertinent positive and negative findings related to the patient's chief complaint.

DIFFERENTIAL DIAGNOSIS

In order of likelihood (with 1 being most likely); list 5 possible diagnoses:

1.

2.

3.

4.

5.

DIAGNOSTIC WORKUP

List immediate plans (up to 5):

1.

2.

3.

4.

5.

PRACTICE CASE 13

Chart Information

Chief complaint: A 35-year-old man comes to the clinic complaining of persistent diarrhea.

Vital signs: T: 37.9 C (100.2 F), BP: 128/92 mm Hg, HR: 80/min, RR: 16/min

History

The diarrhea has been intermittent over the last year. He occasionally has episodes of fecal incontinence, where he finds small amounts of stool in his underwear. The episodes of diarrhea are occasionally associated with some blood, which appears "mixed in" with the stool, and large amounts of mucus. On any given day, the patient may suffer 10 to 20 bowel movements. He has suffered chronic lower abdominal pain, which he rates a 4 on an intensity scale of 1 to 10. The pain is described as "crampy." Additionally, the patient has suffered intermittent fevers, chills, night sweats, and a 20-lb weight loss. He has noticed some intermittent joint pain, but has not suffered any visual changes, red eyes, or skin rash. The joint pain has mainly been in his knees. There are no known sick contacts, and aside from a recent trip to Israel, he has not left the country. Prior to this last year, the patient reports being in good health, although 2 years ago he had a perianal fistula repaired about a year and a half ago. He takes no medications, either prescription or over the counter, takes no dietary supplements, and has no drug allergies. An uncle had some sort of "problem with his gut" requiring surgery and resection, and he now has a fecal waste bag attached to his abdomen. Otherwise, the patient cannot recall any illnesses that run in the family, specifically no gastrointestinal cancer. The patient does not smoke, drink, or use any drugs, and is a full-time rabbinical student. He is sexually active and monogamous with his wife and has two healthy children.

Physical Examination

The patient appears thin and pale but is in no apparent distress. His sclera and conjunctiva appear normal, pupils are equally round and reactive to light, and extra-ocular movements are intact. His chest is clear to auscultation bilaterally. Extremities reveal no cyanosis or clubbing. His cardiac exam demonstrates normal sounds, rate, and rhythm, without any murmurs, rubs, or peripheral edema. On abdominal exam, his liver and spleen are not enlarged. He has normal active bowel sounds, and his abdomen is tympanic to percussion in all four quadrants. He is mildly tender to palpation in the right lower quadrant, but displays no rebound tenderness or guarding. Murphy sign is absent. There are no skin lesions, and his knees appear normal, with no warmth or effusion.

Practice Case 13

Standardized Patient History-Taking Checklist

1.

2.

3.

4.

5.

6.

7.

8.

9.

10.

11.

12.

13.

14.

15.

Standardized Patient Physical Examination Checklist

1.

2.

3.

4.

5.

6.

7.

8.

9.

10.

HISTORY: Include significant positives and negatives from the history of present illness, past medical history, review of system(s), social history, and family history.

PHYSICAL EXAMINATION: Indicate only pertinent positive and negative findings related to the patient's chief complaint.

DIFFERENTIAL DIAGNOSIS

In order of likelihood (with 1 being most likely); list 5 possible diagnoses:

1.

2.

3.

4.

5.

DIAGNOSTIC WORKUP

List immediate plans (up to 5):

1.

2.

3.

4.

5.

PRACTICE CASE 14

Chart Information

Chief complaint: A 22-year-old woman comes to the office complaining of many years of intermittent abdominal pain.

Vital signs: T: 37.0 C (98.6 F), BP: 128/88 mm Hg, HR: 80/min, RR: 14/min

History

The pain has occurred over the last five years and seems to occur intermittently and without warning. It is colicky and diffuse in nature. On a scale of 1 to 10, she rates the pain a four. She has not had any fevers or focal pain, but has had both intermittent diarrhea and constipation and also suffers from bloating and gas. Her main problems are diarrhea and painful bloating, although they have never woken her from sleep. Her stools, while loose, are not of a large volume, do not appear greasy, are not particularly dark, light, or foul smelling, and do not have any obvious blood present. She denies any weight loss, anorexia, joint pains, rash, visual problems, nausea, reflux symptoms, or early satiety. The constipation, when present, can last for days to months. During these periods, she often feels as if she cannot completely evacuate her bowels, even when she does have a bowel movement. Aside from her bowel problems, she reports being generally well and has not suffered from these events as a child or teenager. Occasionally, she needs over-the-counter laxatives and antidiarrhea medication (depending on which is needed), but otherwise does not take any medications. She is allergic to sulfa drugs, vitamin C, and aspirin, all of which give her severe headaches. In the past, she has taken citalopram for depression, her only major past medical problem. She has had no abdominal operations. She states that she has an estranged relationship with her mother and never knew her father and thus does not know what diseases exist in her family history. She neither drinks nor smokes cigarettes, although she uses marijuana recreationally once or twice a month. The patient denies being sexually active currently and has no history of sexually transmitted diseases. Four years ago, she had a normal vaginal delivery of healthy twins.

Physical Examination

The patient is sitting comfortably on the examination table. Her chest is clear to auscultation bilaterally. Her eyes appear normal, with normal pupils and extraocular movements. There is no stare or protrusion. Her thyroid is normal to inspection and palpation. Cardiovascular exam demonstrates normal sounds, rate, and rhythm, without any murmurs, rubs, or gallops. On abdominal exam, percussion and palpation do not reveal an enlarged liver or spleen. She has normal active bowel sounds, and the abdomen is tympanic to percussion in all four quadrants. There is mild tenderness to palpation in all quadrants. No masses are palpable. No Murphy sign is present. Her skin appears normal, without evidence of a rash or other lesions.

Practice Case 14

Standardized Patient History-Taking Checklist

1.

2.

3.

4.

5.

6.

7.

8.

9.

10.

11.

12.

13.

14.

15.

16.

17.

Standardized Patient Physical Examination Checklist

1.

2.

3.

4.

5.

6.

7.

8.

9.

10.

HISTORY: Include significant positives and negatives from the history of present illness, past medical history, review of system(s), social history, and family history.

PHYSICAL EXAMINATION: Indicate only pertinent positive and negative findings related to the patient's chief complaint.

DIFFERENTIAL DIAGNOSIS

In order of likelihood (with 1 being most likely); list 5 possible diagnoses:

1.

2.

3.

4.

5.

DIAGNOSTIC WORKUP

List immediate plans (up to 5):

1.

2.

3.

4.

5.

PRACTICE CASE 15

Chart Information

Chief complaint: A 65-year-old man comes to the clinic complaining of progressive breathlessness.

Vital signs: T: 36.6 C (97.6 F), BP: 130/82 mm Hg, HR: 98/min, RR: 24/min

History

Over the last 1 to 2 years, the patient has suffered from progressive breathlessness, first with exercise, and now even at rest. Prior to this, he has had a dry, hacking cough, which he states he has had since working in construction thirty years ago. This cough has also gotten worse, although he rarely brings up more than some thin, white sputum. Occasionally, he will notice a faint wheeze after a spell of coughing. He denies any chest pain associated with the cough, although he has had a 30-lb weight loss over the past 6 months despite an appetite that has not changed. He has not had any fever, chills, or night sweats and does not know of any sick contacts. The sensation of breathlessness is improved with rest and does not change with position. He is able to sleep at night and has not noticed any lower extremity swelling. Before the last few years, the patient felt he was in good health, although he suffers from hypertension. He takes atenolol for his blood pressure, a daily baby aspirin, and has no known drug allergies. There are no illnesses that run in the patient's family. He is currently a retired widower and enjoys gardening, although this has become nearly impossible due to breathlessness. His construction work mainly involved renovating old buildings, although prior to this, he worked in a ship-building yard and a quarry. He does not drink, has smoked half-a-pack per day for 50 years, and has never used illicit substances.

Physical Examination

The patient appears anxious and mildly uncomfortable and is thin and pale. There are no palpable lymph nodes in the cervical, supraclavicular, or axillary regions. He appears to be breathing at a rate of approximately 25 to 30 breaths/min, and he coughs when asked to breathe deeply or expire fully. He is not using any accessory muscles of respiration, and his chest wall appears symmetrical. His chest is clear to auscultation bilaterally, and tactile fremitus is normal. There is no cyanosis, clubbing, or edema present. His heart demonstrates normal sounds, rate, and rhythm. There were no murmurs, rubs, or gallops present. The point of maximal impulse is not displaced. The top of his jugular venous fluid column appears at approximately 2 cm above his sternoclavicular notch. On abdominal exam, the liver is not enlarged. He has normal active bowel sounds, and the abdomen is tympanic to percussion in all four quadrants with no tenderness on palpation.

Practice Case 15

Standardized Patient History-Taking Checklist

1.

2.

3.

4.

5.

6.

7.

8.

9.

10.

11.

12.

13.

14.

15.

16.

17.

18.

Standardized Patient Physical Examination Checklist

1.

2.

3.

4.

5.

6.

7.

8.

9.

10.

HISTORY: Include significant positives and negatives from the history of present illness, past medical history, review of system(s), social history, and family history.

PHYSICAL EXAMINATION: Indicate only pertinent positive and negative findings related to the patient's chief complaint.

DIFFERENTIAL DIAGNOSIS

In order of likelihood (with 1 being most likely); list 5 possible diagnoses:

1.

2.

3.

4.

5.

DIAGNOSTIC WORKUP

List immediate plans (up to 5):

1.

2.

3.

4.

5.

PRACTICE CASE 16

Chart Information

Chief complaint: An 18-year-old man comes to the emergency department complaining of scrotal pain.

Vital signs: T: 37.3 C (99.1 F), BP: 130/80 mm Hg, HR: 105/min, RR: 22/min

History

The patient is present with his mother. According to the patient, earlier in the evening, about 4 hours ago, the patient woke from sleep with sudden right groin and testicular pain. The pain is rated a 10/10 and is unlike anything the patient has ever felt before. The pain is dull and throbbing and seems to spread from his testicle toward his groin. According to the patient, the testicle appears swollen and red. Since the pain began, the patient has had two episodes of nonbloody emesis and is currently nauseated. He denies any recent dysuria, penile lesions, or discharge, and has had no fever, chills, or diarrhea. The patient does report some stomach cramping and has had some mild pain. He also thinks he has some swelling in his left knee. He reports that he did suffer some trauma to his testicles earlier in the day, while at soccer practice, but that the pain quickly resolved and was nothing like his current pain level. In the last 4 hours, nothing has seemed to affect his pain, although he states that there is slightly less pain if he holds his testicle in his hand. Prior to this, he has been in good health. He has no major illnesses and knows of none that run in his family. He has no allergies and takes no medications. The patient is at first sheepish about discussing his sexual activity. However, once his mother reluctantly leaves the room, he admits to having had sex a number of times with three different female partners. He reports "sometimes" wearing condoms. The patient has, to his knowledge, never had a sexually transmitted disease. The patient denies smoking, drinks rarely at social events (1 to 2 beers over the weekend), and does not use illicit substances.

Physical Examination

The patient is in moderate discomfort and is unable to sit still. His lungs are clear to auscultation bilaterally. On abdominal exam, the liver is not enlarged. He has normal active bowel sounds, and the abdomen is tympanic to percussion in all four quadrants with no tenderness on palpation. Extremities reveal no cyanosis, clubbing, or edema. His knees reveal no effusion or warmth. Skin exam is normal, without any evidence of rash or lesions.

KAPLAN **medical**

Practice Case 16

Standardized Patient History-Taking Checklist

1.

2.

3.

4.

5.

6.

7.

8.

9.

10.

11.

12.

13.

14.

15.

Standardized Patient Physical Examination Checklist

1.

2.

3.

4.

5.

6.

7.

8.

9.

10.

HISTORY: Include significant positives and negatives from the history of present illness, past medical history, review of system(s), social history, and family history.

PHYSICAL EXAMINATION: Indicate only pertinent positive and negative findings related to the patient's chief complaint.

DIFFERENTIAL DIAGNOSIS

In order of likelihood (with 1 being most likely); list 5 possible diagnoses:

1.

2.

3.

4.

5.

DIAGNOSTIC WORKUP

List immediate plans (up to 5):

1.

2.

3.

4.

5.

PRACTICE CASE 17

Chart Information

Chief complaint: A 67-year-old man comes to the emergency department complaining of tearing chest pain.

Vital signs: T: 38.2 C (100.8 F), BP: 195/115 mm Hg, HR: 110/min, RR: 30/min

History

The pain began approximately 1 hour ago, while the patient was sitting and watching television. It is intense, rating a 10/10 on a pain scale, and is described as "sharp and tearing." The pain is located slightly left of the midline of his chest and moves through toward his back. The patient also reports feeling short of breath, anxious, mildly nauseated, and sweaty. Nothing seems to improve or worsen his symptoms; it is not relieved or exacerbated by rest or exertion. The aspirin and acetaminophen he took earlier have provided little relief. Prior to today's events, he has felt ill for about a week. He has noticed intermittent, mild chest pain, a worsening dry cough, and has had difficulty swallowing his food. He denies any recent fevers, chills, weight changes, swelling, orthopnea, or urinary or gastrointestinal symptoms. These symptoms are similar to a heart attack he had two years ago, but today's pain is much worse. The patient is not allergic to any medications and takes aspirin, atenolol, atorvastatin, and hydrochlorothiazide. He suffers from coronary artery disease, having had a heart attack 2 years ago, and has also been diagnosed with hypertension and high cholesterol. He denies having diabetes and does not think it runs in his family. Indeed, he states that his family is very healthy, and he specifically denies any family history of heart disease. He smokes one to two packs of cigarettes a day, and has done so since age 17. He does not drink or use drugs and has a healthy diet. Currently, the patient is not sexually active but was "quite a stallion" when he served in the Navy. He reports a history of syphilis and gonorrhea in the distant past.

Physical Examination

The patient appears anxious and uncomfortable. His chest is clear to auscultation and percussion, and tactile fremitus is normal. Tenderness is not reproduced by palpation. Cardiac exam demonstrates normal sounds, rate, and rhythm, without any murmurs, rubs, or gallops. The top of his internal jugular venous column is present at about 2 to 3 cm above the sternal notch. No carotid bruits are heard. His point of maximal impulse is normal in size and location. His pulses are normal in both upper extremities, and his carotid pulse has a normal upstroke and amplitude. On abdominal exam, the liver is not enlarged. He has normal active bowel sounds, and his abdomen is tympanic to percussion in all four quadrants with no tenderness on deep palpation. Extremities reveal 2+ bilateral pedal pulses, no cyanosis, clubbing, or edema. The lower extremity motor and sensory function is intact.

Practice Case 17

Standardized Patient History-Taking Checklist

1.

2.

3.

4.

5.

6.

7.

8.

9.

10.

11.

12.

13.

14.

Standardized Patient Physical Examination Checklist

1.

2.

3.

4.

5.

6.

7.

8.

9.

10.

11.

12.

HISTORY: Include significant positives and negatives from the history of present illness, past medical history, review of system(s), social history, and family history.

PHYSICAL EXAMINATION: Indicate only pertinent positive and negative findings related to the patient's chief complaint.

DIFFERENTIAL DIAGNOSIS

In order of likelihood (with 1 being most likely); list 5 possible diagnoses:

1.

2.

3.

4.

5.

DIAGNOSTIC WORKUP

List immediate plans (up to 5):

1.

2.

3.

4.

5.

PRACTICE CASE 18

Chart Information

Chief complaint: A 43-year-old woman comes to the clinic complaining of dizziness.

Vital signs: T: 37.0 C (98.6 F), BP: 128/84 mm Hg, HR: 50/min, RR: 14/min

History

Over the last 6 months, the patient has had episodes of dizziness. She describes feeling unsteady on her feet and having the room spin about her. These spells can last from 20 minutes to hours and do not have a clear precipitating factor. Additionally, she has suffered from fluctuating hearing loss and often has difficulty understanding what people are saying. She thinks her left ear is worse and describes a sensation of fullness in that ear. The patient also reports a low-pitched "buzz" heard predominantly in the left ear. She denies any fevers, chills, head trauma, headaches, seizure-like activity, nausea, or changes in weight or appetite. She has not found anything that helps her symptoms, but she thinks they may be slightly worse with position changes. Aside from these symptoms, which have never bothered her before, she has been relatively healthy. She does suffer from hypertension and takes atenolol for this condition, as well as a daily aspirin. The patient also has a history of depression, but states she is currently "okay" and not suicidal. She has no drug allergies. Her family history is unremarkable. She does not drink, smoke, or use illicit substances and reports regular exercise and a healthy diet.

Physical Examination

The patient is sitting comfortably on the examination table and is alert and oriented to person, place, and date. Her head appears and feels normal. Her extraocular movements are intact, and her pupils are round and reactive to light. She has mild inducible nystagmus on extremes of gaze. Her ears appear normal; there is no obstructions in either external auditory canal, and the tympanic membranes are clearly visualized. There is no pain with movement of the pinna. Her nose, throat, and mouth appear normal. The nasal turbinates are not congested; there is no tonsillar enlargement, exudates, or erythema; and there are no ulcers, vesicles, or other lesions. Her neck is supple, without thyroid or cervical lymph-node enlargement. The patient's cranial nerves are intact to gross exam. The tuning fork exam is as follows: When the tuning fork is placed on the bridge of the forehead, the sound is described as louder in her right ear. When the tuning fork is placed first behind the mastoid then near the ear (to test bone and air conduction), air conduction is greater than bone conduction, particularly in the right ear. She has a normal gait, performs a finger-to-nose test well, and does not have a Romberg sign. Her motor strength is normal in all muscle groups, as is her sensation. Deep tendon reflexes are normal. Her toes are downgoing when the sole of her foot is rubbed with the reflex hammer. There are no carotid bruits upon auscultation. Auscultation of the patient's chest reveals a normal cardiac exam; heart sounds are normal, with no murmurs, rubs, or gallops present.

Practice Case 18

Standardized Patient History-Taking Checklist

1.

2.

3.

4.

5.

6.

7.

8.

9.

10.

11.

12.

13.

14.

Standardized Patient Physical Examination Checklist

1.

2.

3.

4.

5.

6.

7.

8.

9.

10.

11.

12.

13.

14.

15.

16.

HISTORY: Include significant positives and negatives from the history of present illness, past medical history, review of system(s), social history, and family history.

PHYSICAL EXAMINATION: Indicate only pertinent positive and negative findings related to the patient's chief complaint.

DIFFERENTIAL DIAGNOSIS

In order of likelihood (with 1 being most likely); list 5 possible diagnoses:

1.

2.

3.

4.

5.

DIAGNOSTIC WORKUP

List immediate plans (up to 5):

1.

2.

3.

4.

5.

PRACTICE CASE 19

Chart Information

Chief complaint: A 47-year-old man comes to the clinic complaining of nausea, fatigue, and yellow skin.

Vital signs: T: 37.1 C (98.8 F), BP: 118/72 mm Hg, HR: 95/min, RR: 14/min

History

Over the last year, the patient has gradually developed increasing fatigue, intermittent nausea (although no emesis), and right upper quadrant pain. Further, over the last week, his urine has turned tea-colored. He states he has been a heavy drinker for the last five to ten years and knows his problems might be related to his alcohol. He just finished a week-long binge, with his last drink occurring yesterday afternoon. His pain is constant and dull, does not radiate, and is rated a 4/10 on a pain scale. In addition to his current symptoms, he has had some joint pains in his knees and elbows for the past week, but denies any rash, visual changes, fevers, chills, or changes in his bowel movements. Nothing seems to make his symptoms better or worse, although the large amounts of acetaminophen he has taken over the last week seem to help his joint pain. He has suffered from mild anorexia, preferring to drink rather than eat, and has lost at least 20 lb over the past 2 months. Prior to his alcoholism, the patient reports being healthy, has no drug allergies, and does not take any medications. His family is fairly healthy, although he knows of an uncle who died of "some liver problem." He is currently unemployed and lives in a homeless shelter. He is not currently sexually active but has had numerous partners in the past, does not use condoms regularly, and has a history of gonorrhea. The patient denies current tobacco or drug use, but states he used to inject heroin.

Physical Examination

The patient appears comfortable, although he is gaunt and has yellow-tinged skin. His chest is clear to auscultation bilaterally. His heart demonstrates normal sounds, rate, and rhythm. There are no murmurs, rubs, or gallops. On abdominal exam, his abdomen appears nondistended, and there is no bulging of the flanks. The patient is moderately tender in the right upper quadrant to palpation and percussion, but does not appear to have an enlarged liver or spleen. Although the patient does have a tender right upper quadrant, no Murphy sign can be elicited. There is no shifting dullness or fluid wave present. He has normal active bowel sounds, and his abdomen is tympanic to percussion in all four quadrants. His extremities show no cyanosis, clubbing, or edema, and his joints are cool to the touch, without evidence of effusions. An examination of his skin reveals two tattoos, which the patient reports getting done in prison, but no spider angiomas, palmar erythema, gynecomastia, or other signs of liver disease.

Practice Case 19

Standardized Patient History-Taking Checklist

1.

2.

3.

4.

5.

6.

7.

8.

9.

10.

11.

12.

13.

14.

15.

16.

Standardized Patient Physical Examination Checklist

1.

2.

3.

4.

5.

6.

7.

8.

9.

10.

11.

HISTORY: Include significant positives and negatives from the history of present illness, past medical history, review of system(s), social history, and family history.

PHYSICAL EXAMINATION: Indicate only pertinent positive and negative findings related to the patient's chief complaint.

DIFFERENTIAL DIAGNOSIS

In order of likelihood (with 1 being most likely); list 5 possible diagnoses:

1.

2.

3.

4.

5.

DIAGNOSTIC WORKUP

List immediate plans (up to 5):

1.

2.

3.

4.

5.

PRACTICE CASE 20

Chart Information

Chief complaint: A 66-year-old woman comes to the urgent care clinic after an episode of loss of consciousness.

Vital signs: T: 37.0 C (98.6 F), BP: 118/70 mm Hg, HR: 50/min, RR: 14/min

History

This morning, while doing housework, the patient suffered a brief loss of consciousness. She is not sure exactly what happened—she had been hard at work scrubbing the floor and, when she arose, suddenly felt light-headed and then just "blacked out." She arose less than 30 seconds later according to the clock on the kitchen wall. For a few minutes, she felt nauseated, but then recovered. She does not think she hit her head. Just prior to falling, she felt slightly sick to her stomach and was mildly confused when she woke, although she denies bowel or bladder incontinence, tongue biting, or prolonged confusion. The patient did not suffer any chest pain or chest tightness, although she does occasionally have palpitations. She denies any shortness of breath. The last episode of palpitations was earlier that morning. She cannot think of any clear precipitating factors. The patient has a history of hypertension, diabetes, and coronary artery disease and had a heart attack about 5 years ago, but denies having a seizure or a previous syncopal or near-syncopal episode. She currently takes aspirin, atenolol, metformin, and lisinopril. Heart disease and diabetes run in her family, and both of her parents died from heart attacks in their fifties. She smokes about half a pack of cigarettes a day and has done so since age 20, but does not drink or use illicit drugs. Currently, she is employed as a schoolteacher and lives with her husband of 40 years.

Physical Examination

The patient is comfortably sitting on the examination table and is alert and oriented to person, place, and time, displaying good concentration and cooperation with the exam. The patient's head is normocephalic and atraumatic. Her chest is clear to auscultation bilaterally. Her heart demonstrates normal sounds, rate, and rhythm with no murmurs, rubs, or gallops. There are no carotid bruits, and the top of her jugular venous column is about 1 cm above the sternal notch. Her point of maximal impulse is normal in size, location, and intensity. On abdominal exam, her liver is not enlarged and her abdomen is tympanic to percussion in all four quadrants. There is no tenderness to palpation, and no masses are present. Her cranial nerves are intact. Muscle strength is 5/5 in all extremities, and sensation is intact to pinprick and light touch. Deep tendon reflexes are normal, and her toes are downgoing when the bottom of her foot is rubbed with your reflex hammer. She has a normal gait and no evidence of a Romberg sign.

Practice Case 20

Standardized Patient History-Taking Checklist

1.

2.

3.

4.

5.

6.

7.

8.

9.

10.

11.

12.

13.

14.

15.

Standardized Patient Physical Examination Checklist

1.

2.

3.

4.

5.

6.

7.

8.

9.

10.

11.

12.

13.

HISTORY: Include significant positives and negatives from the history of present illness, past medical history, review of system(s), social history, and family history.

PHYSICAL EXAMINATION: Indicate only pertinent positive and negative findings related to the patient's chief complaint.

DIFFERENTIAL DIAGNOSIS	DIAGNOSTIC WORKUP
In order of likelihood (with 1 being most likely); list 5 possible diagnoses:	List immediate plans (up to 5):
1.	1.
2.	2.
3.	3.
4.	4.
5.	5.

PRACTICE CASE 21

Chart Information

Chief complaint: A 66-year-old man comes to the clinic complaining of a cough and fever.

Vital signs: T: 38.3 C (101.0 F), BP: 146/90 mm Hg, HR: 107/min, RR: 28/min

History

Although the patient has a 2-year history of a fairly constant, productive cough, over the last 3 days his symptoms have worsened. His phlegm has turned greenish-yellow and foul smelling and his cough, which usually bothers him mainly early in the morning and late at night, is now constant throughout the day. He has been running some low-grade fevers, although he has not suffered any chills, night-sweats, chest pain, palpitations, or nausea. Intermittently, he has noticed some fleeting chest tightness and wheezing. The patient has noticed some small streaks of blood in his sputum, but denies any frank bleeding. Prior to this event, he reports feeling generally fatigued and having a 10- to 20-lb weight loss over the past few months. He has no medication allergies and currently takes atenolol, warfarin, and uses an ipratropium inhaler. He uses these medications as prescribed and has not missed or doubled any recent doses. Over the past couple of years, he has suffered from two episodes of pneumonia requiring hospitalization, a pulmonary embolus, chronic obstructive pulmonary disease, and high blood pressure. He does not know of any illnesses that run in his family. The patient does not smoke, having quit 3 days ago. Prior to this, he smoked a pack of cigarettes a day for the past 40 years. He does not drink or use any illicit substances and is a retired postal employee.

Physical Examination

The patient appears anxious and mildly uncomfortable. He is thin and pale and is leaning forward, with arms resting on his knees. There are no palpable lymph nodes in the cervical, supraclavicular, or axillary regions. He appears to be breathing at a rate of approximately 25 to 30 breaths/min and coughs when asked to breathe deeply or expire fully. He is not using any accessory muscles of respiration, and his chest wall appears symmetrical. His chest is clear to auscultation bilaterally, and tactile fremitus is normal. There is no cyanosis, clubbing, or edema present. His heart demonstrates normal sounds, rate, and rhythm. There were no murmurs, rubs, or gallops present. The point of maximal impulse is not displaced. The top of his jugular venous fluid column appears at approximately 2 cm above his sternoclavicular notch. On abdominal exam, the liver is not enlarged. He has normal active bowel sounds, and the abdomen is tympanic to percussion in all four quadrants with no tenderness on palpation.

Practice Case 21

Standardized Patient History-Taking Checklist

1.

2.

3.

4.

5.

6.

7.

8.

9.

10.

11.

12.

13.

14.

15.

16.

17.

18.

Standardized Patient Physical Examination Checklist

1.

2.

3.

4.

5.

6.

7.

8.

9.

10.

HISTORY: Include significant positives and negatives from the history of present illness, past medical history, review of system(s), social history, and family history.

PHYSICAL EXAMINATION: Indicate only pertinent positive and negative findings related to the patient's chief complaint.

DIFFERENTIAL DIAGNOSIS

In order of likelihood (with 1 being most likely); list 5 possible diagnoses:

1.

2.

3.

4.

5.

DIAGNOSTIC WORKUP

List immediate plans (up to 5):

1.

2.

3.

4.

5.

PRACTICE CASE 22

Chart Information

Chief complaint: A 51-year-old man comes to the office complaining of abdominal pain.

Vital signs: T: 37 C (98.6 F), BP: 138/85 mm Hg, HR: 88/min, RR: 14/min

History

For the last three months, the patient has suffered a dull, midepigastric pain. The pain is located in the center of his stomach and seems to spread through to his back. It is rated a 4–5/10, but is constant and, despite its insidious onset, seems to be getting worse. It is not related to exertion, although the patient states he has been too exhausted to do much of anything recently. It is slightly improved with sitting forward and made slightly worse by lying flat. Additionally, the patient reports a 15-lb weight loss over the last month and a loss of appetite. Eating seems to make the pain slightly worse. Also, when the patient does eat, he reports feeling full quickly. The patient also reports being told that he has yellow eyes, although he has not noticed this. He denies any fevers, nausea, reflux symptoms, chest pain, changes in bowel habits, or urinary symptoms. He takes no medications, prescriptions or otherwise, and specifically denies taking any nonsteroidal anti-inflammatory medications. His past medical history is remarkable for a case of idiopathic pancreatitis earlier this year, superficial thrombophlebitis while hospitalized for pancreatitis, and borderline hyperglycemia (currently diet controlled), but he has never had anything that felt like his current condition. He knows of no illnesses that run in the family, specifically no malignancies or gastrointestinal illnesses. The patient sheepishly admits to smoking a "pack or two" a day for the last 30 years but drinks only rarely (1 to 3 beers during the weekend). He denies using any illicit substances.

Physical Examination

The patient has no cervical, supraclavicular, or axillary lymphadenopathy. His sclerae are icteric. His chest is clear to auscultation bilaterally, and tactile fremitus is within normal limits. His cardiac exam demonstrates normal sounds, rate, and rhythm, without any murmurs, rubs, or peripheral edema. His jugular venous pressure is about 7 cm H_2O. On abdominal exam, his liver and spleen are not enlarged. He has normal active bowel sounds, and his abdomen is tympanic to percussion in all four quadrants. He is mildly tender to palpation in the midepigastric area, but displays no rebound tenderness or guarding. He has a negative Murphy sign and a nonpalpable gallbladder. No masses are present. His skin shows no sign of rash or other lesions.

Practice Case 22

Standardized Patient History-Taking Checklist

1.

2.

3.

4.

5.

6.

7.

8.

9.

10.

11.

12.

13.

14.

Standardized Patient Physical Examination Checklist

1.

2.

3.

4.

5.

6.

7.

8.

9.

10.

11.

12.

HISTORY: Include significant positives and negatives from the history of present illness, past medical history, review of system(s), social history, and family history.

PHYSICAL EXAMINATION: Indicate only pertinent positive and negative findings related to the patient's chief complaint.

DIFFERENTIAL DIAGNOSIS

In order of likelihood (with 1 being most likely); list 5 possible diagnoses:

1.

2.

3.

4.

5.

DIAGNOSTIC WORKUP

List immediate plans (up to 5):

1.

2.

3.

4.

5.

PRACTICE CASE 23

Chart Information

Chief complaint: A 60-year-old man comes to the clinic complaining of blood in his urine.

Vital signs: T: 37 C (98.6 F), BP: 118/70 mm Hg, HR: 62/min, RR: 14/min

History

Over the last 3 months, there have been three episodes of bright red, bloody urine. There are no clear precipitating factors, and the blood seems to persist throughout the stream of urine. The patient denies any pain specifically associated with the bloody urine, but does report having some episodes of "burning" when he urinates. Additionally, he has been frequently using the bathroom (at least once an hour) over the last few months, and he often feels he cannot hold his urine until he gets to the restroom. During the night, the patient will wake four to five times needing to use the bathroom. He denies any other pain, anorexia, fever, chills, weight loss, flank pain, or previous episodes of bleeding. He is not aware of anything that makes his symptoms better or worse. Prior to this, the patient reports being healthy; indeed, he runs five to ten miles at least 4 days a week. He has no allergies or other medical problems and, aside from a daily aspirin, takes no medications. He did have one extremely painful kidney stone 5 years prior, but has not had any urinary tract infections or other episodes of stones. He has not had any dietary changes or gastrointestinal symptoms. There are no diseases that run in the family, specifically no cancer that the patient knows of. The patient does not drink, smoke cigarettes, or use any illicit substances. He denies any history of STDs, is monogamous, and is currently sexually active with his wife of 35 years. The patient works as a patent lawyer and has done so for the last 32 years.

Physical Examination

The patient appears comfortable and in no apparent distress. His chest is clear to auscultation bilaterally. Cardiac examination reveals normal heart sounds, rate, and rhythm. There are no murmurs, rubs, or gallops. His extremities show no evidence of cyanosis, clubbing, or edema. The abdomen is tympanic in all four quadrants. He has normal active bowel sounds. There are no palpable masses, and the abdomen is nontender and nondistended. No surgical scars are present. There is no costovertebral angle tenderness, and there is no skin lesions.

Practice Case 23

Standardized Patient History-Taking Checklist

1.

2.

3.

4.

5.

6.

7.

8.

9.

10.

11.

12.

13.

14.

15.

16.

Standardized Patient Physical Examination Checklist

1.

2.

3.

4.

5.

6.

7.

8.

HISTORY: Include significant positives and negatives from the history of present illness, past medical history, review of system(s), social history, and family history.

PHYSICAL EXAMINATION: Indicate only pertinent positive and negative findings related to the patient's chief complaint.

DIFFERENTIAL DIAGNOSIS

In order of likelihood (with 1 being most likely); list 5 possible diagnoses:

1.

2.

3.

4.

5.

DIAGNOSTIC WORKUP

List immediate plans (up to 5):

1.

2.

3.

4.

5.

PRACTICE CASE 24

Chart Information

Chief complaint: A 24-year-old woman comes to the office complaining of weakness.

Vital signs: T: 37.2 C (98.9 F), BP: 115/77 mm Hg, HR: 67/min, RR: 16/min

History

Gradually, over the past 2 months, the patient has felt increasingly fatigued. The fatigue is constant, and she has trouble localizing any specific weakness, soreness, or pain. She has, however, noticed episodes of blurry and double vision, particularly when walking up or down the stairs in her house. Additionally, she occasionally, over the last week, has become "exhausted" when eating a meal. Her tongue and jaw become weak, and she has difficulty chewing and swallowing, although there is no pain. In general, she feels that everything she does tires her out. Nothing seems to improve her symptoms. This has never happened before, and she is worried that she might fall when using the stairs. Further, she feels her symptoms are getting worse. She denies any rash, fever, chills, joint pains, recent illnesses, or seizure-like activity. She has not had any heat or cold intolerance, palpitations, diarrhea, constipation, dysuria, or urinary frequency and reports being generally healthy and in a good mood. She has no drug allergies, and, aside from a birth control pill, takes no medications. The patient has a normal appetite and has not lost weight. Her family history is significant for a mother with "some neck gland problem," but is otherwise unremarkable. She does not smoke, drink, or use illicit substances and is currently a mechanical engineering graduate student.

Physical Examination

The patient appears healthy, is in no apparent distress, and is alert and oriented to person, place, and time. Her extraocular muscles are intact, and there is no inducible ptosis or other evidence of bulbar fatigue. Pupils are equally round and reactive to light. Her thyroid gland is not palpably enlarged, and she has no cervical, supraclavicular, or axillary lymphadenopathy. The patient's chest is clear to auscultation bilaterally. Cardiac exam reveals normal heart sounds, without evidence of murmurs, rubs, or gallops. Her abdomen is soft, nontender, and nondistended, without any palpable masses or visible scars. There is no hepatosplenomegaly, and her abdomen is tympanic to percussion in all four quadrants. The patient's cranial nerves II though XII are intact, and her muscle strength and cutaneous sensation are normal. Deep tendon reflexes are normal, and her toes, when her foot is stroked with the reflex hammer, are downgoing.

Practice Case 24

Standardized Patient History-Taking Checklist

1.

2.

3.

4.

5.

6.

7.

8.

9.

10.

11.

12.

13.

14.

15.

16.

Standardized Patient Physical Examination Checklist

1.

2.

3.

4.

5.

6.

7.

8.

9.

10.

11.

12.

13.

14.

HISTORY: Include significant positives and negatives from the history of present illness, past medical history, review of system(s), social history, and family history.

PHYSICAL EXAMINATION: Indicate only pertinent positive and negative findings related to the patient's chief complaint.

DIFFERENTIAL DIAGNOSIS	**DIAGNOSTIC WORKUP**
In order of likelihood (with 1 being most likely); list 5 possible diagnoses:	List immediate plans (up to 5):

1.	1.
2.	2.
3.	3.
4.	4.
5.	5.

PRACTICE CASE 25

Chart Information

Chief complaint: A 68-year-old man comes to the clinic complaining of inability to have sex with his wife.

Vital signs: T: 37.2 C (99.0 F), BP: 130/78 mm Hg, HR: 62/min, RR: 14/min

History

The patient initially does not wish to discuss his problem and requests a prescription for the "little blue pill" so he can "get out of here." After some coaxing, he reports that for the last 8 months, he has been unable to have sex with his wife. The onset of his problem has been gradual, progressive, and constant. He is able to get an erection sometimes, but has difficulty maintaining it; he also has some difficulty and occasional pain ejaculating. The patient is still interested in sex and attracted to his wife, although he admits he does not have the same drive he used to. He does not masturbate and is uncertain if he has nocturnal or morning erections. He denies any dysuria, testicular or penile pain, penile discharge, breast enlargement or discharge, or visual changes and reports good relations with his wife. He has had some fatigue and reports some constipation, but otherwise has not noted any change in his health status. He has not had any heat or cold intolerance. The patient has been under some stress, as his son is getting divorced, but denies depressed mood, sleep disturbances, or disinterest in pleasurable activities. He has not noticed anything that improves or worsens his symptoms. Prior to these last eight months, the patient reports being in "okay" health and has never had this problem before. He does, however, suffer from diabetes, diagnosed at age 60, high blood pressure, and coronary artery disease, with a myocardial infarction 1 year ago. He is extremely worried about his heart condition and fears having another heart attack. He is currently taking a daily aspirin, metoprolol, metformin, and lisinopril and is not allergic to any medications. His family history includes a father who died of a heart attack in his sixties and a mother with diabetes. The patient currently smokes, although he is now down to half-a-pack a day, after smoking a pack a day for 50 years. He drinks "one or two highballs" a day, but denies ever using any illicit drugs. He has never had any sexually transmitted diseases and reports being monogamous with his wife of 40 years.

Physical Examination

The patient appears comfortable and in no apparent distress. Confrontational visual field testing does not reveal any defects. Funduscopic examination is normal. There is no evidence of an enlarged thyroid. His chest is clear to auscultation bilaterally. Examination and palpation of the chest wall does not reveal any breast enlargement, tenderness, or nipple discharge. Cardiac examination reveals normal heart sounds, rate, and rhythm. There are no murmurs, rubs, or gallops. Pulses are normal in the upper and lower extremities. There are no carotid or abdominal bruits present. His extremities show no evidence of cyanosis, clubbing, edema, lower-extremity wasting, lesions or ulcerations of the feet, or reduced distal sensation to sharp or dull stimuli. On abdominal exam, there is no evidence of hepatosplenomegaly, and the abdomen is tympanic in all four quadrants. He has normal active bowel sounds and is not tender on palpation. No abdominal masses are present.

Practice Case 25

Standardized Patient History-Taking Checklist

1.
2.
3.
4.
5.
6.
7.
8.
9.
10.
11.
12.
13.
14.
15.
16.
17.
18.
19.
20.

Standardized Patient Physical Examination Checklist

1.
2.
3.
4.
5.
6.
7.
8.
9.
10.
11.
12.
13.
14.

KAPLAN
medical

HISTORY: Include significant positives and negatives from the history of present illness, past medical history, review of system(s), social history, and family history.

PHYSICAL EXAMINATION: Indicate only pertinent positive and negative findings related to the patient's chief complaint.

DIFFERENTIAL DIAGNOSIS

In order of likelihood (with 1 being most likely); list 5 possible diagnoses:

1.

2.

3.

4.

5.

DIAGNOSTIC WORKUP

List immediate plans (up to 5):

1.

2.

3.

4.

5.

PRACTICE CASE 26

Chart Information

Chief complaint: A 62-year-old woman comes to the urgent care clinic because of headaches, jaw pain, and occasional vision problems.

Vital signs: T: 38.2 C (100.8 F), BP: 158/70 mm Hg, HR: 66/min, RR: 16/min

History

For the last 6 months, the patient reports having left-sided headaches. Their onset is quick, painful (6/10), and without warning. The pain may sharp or dull and throbbing, but seems to be getting worse. When the attacks occur, which is now almost daily, with episodes lasting up to an hour, the pain quickly reaches its maximum level of intensity. The pain sometimes spreads to the front of her head and sometime to the nape of her neck. Movement, position, and exercise occasionally make the headache slightly worse, but there are no clear triggers or major aggravating factors. Associated with the headaches, the patient has had two episodes of left-sided visual loss, which she describes as a "complete blackout" in the affected eye. Further, over the last three months, when she eats, she will often get pain on the left side of her face. The pain is dull and associated with jaw movement and chewing. She also reports low-grade fevers, a 15-lb weight loss, and a general sense of fatigue and malaise, although no focal weakness. She denies any joint pain, nausea, halos, pain from bright lights, or aura and reports compliance with her medications. She has been taking over-the-counter aspirin and acetaminophen for her headaches, which provides some minimal relief. The patient also takes metoprolol and nitroglycerin as needed for coronary artery disease, hypertension, and anginal symptoms. She has no known drug allergies. She has a mother with migraines, although she herself has not suffered from headaches previously. The patient denies use of alcohol, tobacco, or illicit substances. She works as a corporate lawyer and reports that her stress level, while high, has been manageable and that she is in good spirits despite her ailment.

Physical Examination

The patient is pale and appears ill. She is alert and oriented to person, place, and time and displays good concentration and cooperation with the exam. Her head is normocephalic and atraumatic, but tender to palpation on the left side, in the area anterior to her auricle. There are no palpable cords, temporomandibular joint tenderness, or tenderness with movement of the pinnae. Extraocular movements are intact; pupils are equal, round, and reactive to light; and a funduscopic examination is normal. Otoscopic examination reveals normal-appearing tympanic membranes. Her neck is supple, with no evidence of cervical, supraclavicular, or axillary lymphadenopathy. Cardiac examination reveals normal heart sounds, rate, and rhythm. There are no murmurs, rubs, or gallops. There is no evidence of a carotid or cranial bruit. Extremities show no evidence of cyanosis, clubbing, or edema, and have a full active and passive range of motion. On abdominal exam, there is no evidence of hepatosplenomegaly, and the abdomen is tympanic in all four quadrants. She has normal active bowel sounds and is not tender on palpation. No abdominal masses are present. Cranial nerves II through XII are intact, and muscle strength and sensation are normal in all muscle groups. There is no evidence of muscle wasting or tenderness. Deep tendon reflexes are normal. The patient is able to get up from a seated position and walk in tandem without assistance. She has a normal finger-to-nose test, and does not have Romberg, Brudzinski, or Babinski signs.

Practice Case 26

Standardized Patient History-Taking Checklist

1.

2.

3.

4.

5.

6.

7.

8.

9.

10.

11.

12.

13.

14.

15.

16.

Standardized Patient Physical Examination Checklist

1.

2.

3.

4.

5.

6.

7.

8.

9.

10.

11.

12.

13.

14.

15.

16.

HISTORY: Include significant positives and negatives from the history of present illness, past medical history, review of system(s), social history, and family history.

PHYSICAL EXAMINATION: Indicate only pertinent positive and negative findings related to the patient's chief complaint.

DIFFERENTIAL DIAGNOSIS	DIAGNOSTIC WORKUP
In order of likelihood (with 1 being most likely); list 5 possible diagnoses:	List immediate plans (up to 5):
1.	1.
2.	2.
3.	3.
4.	4.
5.	5.

PRACTICE CASE 27

Chart Information

Chief complaint: A 30-year-old woman comes to the clinic complaining of a vaginal discharge.

Vital signs: T: 37.1 C (98.8 F), BP: 126/70 mm Hg, HR: 68/min, RR: 14/min

History

The discharge started fairly quickly about a week ago. Over the course of 2 days, the patient noticed the occasional presence of a thick, almost frothy-appearing vaginal discharge. The discharge varies in color from green to greenish-white to yellow. The patient reports thinking that she may have seen some blood, but she is not certain. The patient is embarrassed by the itch-iness and the odor, which she states is foul and mildly "fishy." Further, she has had a sense of fullness in her uterus, which also started about a week ago. She denies any weight loss, pelvic pain, fatigue, rash, or previous episodes of discharge or sexually transmitted diseases. She does, however, think she may have had some low-grade fevers over the past week. The patient cannot think of any precipitating event, although she did recently start using a new brand of tampons and wonders if that could be the cause of her symptoms. Nothing seems to improve or worsen her symptoms. She has no drug allergies and takes subcutaneous NPH and regular insulin twice a day. Aside from diabetes and one episode of diabetic ketoacidosis two years ago, she reports having no medical problems. Her family history is unremarkable; both of her parents and her sister are alive and well, without any chronic illnesses. She has never been pregnant, has normal menstrual periods with her last one occurring 2 weeks ago, and is currently sexually active with her boyfriend. She reports using condoms "most of the time." She has never had a Pap smear and cannot remember the last time she had a gynecologic exam. The patient does not smoke, drinks alcohol only rarely, and denies any drug use.

Physical Examination

The patient appears healthy and in no apparent distress. Her chest is clear to auscultation bilater-ally. Cardiovascular exam demonstrates normal sounds, rate and rhythm, without any murmurs, rubs, or gallops. On abdominal exam, she has normal active bowel sounds, and the abdomen is tympanic to percussion in all four quadrants. No masses are palpable. Her skin appears normal, without evidence of a rash or other lesions.

Practice Case 27

Standardized Patient History-Taking Checklist

1.

2.

3.

4.

5.

6.

7.

8.

9.

10.

11.

12.

13.

14.

15.

16.

17.

18.

Standardized Patient Physical Examination Checklist

1.

2.

3.

4.

5.

6.

HISTORY: Include significant positives and negatives from the history of present illness, past medical history, review of system(s), social history, and family history.

PHYSICAL EXAMINATION: Indicate only pertinent positive and negative findings related to the patient's chief complaint.

DIFFERENTIAL DIAGNOSIS

In order of likelihood (with 1 being most likely); list 5 possible diagnoses:

1.

2.

3.

4.

5.

DIAGNOSTIC WORKUP

List immediate plans (up to 5):

1.

2.

3.

4.

5.

PRACTICE CASE 28

Chart Information

Chief complaint: A 22-year-old woman comes to the clinic because of difficulty sleeping.

Vital signs: T: 37.3 C (99.1 F), BP: 128/77 mm Hg, HR: 84/min, RR: 16/min

History

The patient states that she does not really think she needs to see a doctor, but decided to come anyway, as friends and family were insistent. For the past 2 weeks, she has had trouble with her heart and mind racing. Her newfound energy has allowed her to be incredibly productive at work, producing report after report in record time. Unfortunately, few coworkers appreciate her remarkable insights and have pointed out that her reports are "gibberish" and a "word soup." In any case, she has rewarded herself well with a Versace shopping spree and a handful of new credit cards. She feels "spectacular," although she admits that perhaps it is unusual to not need any sleep and wonders if she should take any medication for her sleeping disorder. She denies any fevers, heat or cold intolerance, hair loss, skin changes, hearing voices or seeing visions, or changes in bowel or bladder habits. She has never had these symptoms before, although her past medical history is significant for a major depressive episode treated 4 years ago, as well as occasional episodes of palpitations and excessive sweating. She takes no medications, has no known drug allergies, and knows of no illnesses or psychiatric disorders or symptoms that run in her family. The patient denies any history of recent drug use, but reports that she has been "clubbing" every night these past two weeks with some new boyfriends to celebrate her successes at work. She rarely smokes, but drinks energy drinks mixed with vodka when out with friends. She is not sure how much she drinks and does not wish to discuss that issue. The patient continues to talk excessively, and you have to ask her to stop so that you may refocus the discussion.

Physical/Mental Status Exam

The patient appears well groomed but is obviously agitated and has difficulty sitting still. She is alert and oriented to person, place, and time. Her speech is pressured, but fluid and goal directed. She has no memory defects, either recent or remote, and her attention and concentration are good, as tested by serial sevens. Her mood is euphoric, and her affect is consistent. She does not have any hallucinations, delusions, or paranoias. She denies any wish to hurt herself or others, but has a poor understanding of her condition or its implications. Inspection and palpation of her thyroid gland reveal no goiter. Her chest is clear to auscultation bilaterally. Cardiovascular exam demonstrates normal sounds, rate and rhythm, without any murmurs, rubs, or gallops. On abdominal exam, percussion and palpation do not reveal an enlarged liver or spleen. She has normal active bowel sounds, and the abdomen is tympanic to percussion in all four quadrants. Her skin appears normal, without evidence of a rash or other lesions.

Practice Case 28

Standardized Patient History-Taking Checklist

1.

2.

3.

4.

5.

6.

7.

8.

9.

10.

11.

12.

13.

14.

15.

Standardized Patient Physical Examination Checklist

1.

2.

3.

4.

5.

6.

7.

8.

9.

10.

11.

12.

13.

14.

HISTORY: Include significant positives and negatives from the history of present illness, past medical history, review of system(s), social history, and family history.

PHYSICAL EXAMINATION: Indicate only pertinent positive and negative findings related to the patient's chief complaint.

DIFFERENTIAL DIAGNOSIS

In order of likelihood (with 1 being most likely); list 5 possible diagnoses:

1.

2.

3.

4.

5.

DIAGNOSTIC WORKUP

List immediate plans (up to 5):

1.

2.

3.

4.

5.

PRACTICE CASE 29

Chart Information

Chief complaint: A mother has a 1-year-old child with diarrhea.

Vital signs: Child not available for physical exam.

History

The mother is quite worried, as her 1-year-old son has had a 3-day history of watery diarrhea, as well as episodes of nonbloody greenish-appearing vomiting. The child's diapers are constantly full of watery, loose stool, and the mother thinks she may at one point have seen some blood and mucus. The mother has difficulty quantifying the amount of stool, but finds it hard to believe that such a small child can produce so much foul-smelling stool. She is giving the child oral rehydration solution to keep up with fluid losses, but is worried that her child might need intravenous fluids. In addition, the child has had a low-grade temperature and has been extremely irritable. Several of the child's daycare playmates have also become ill, although no one in the family is affected. She denies noticing a rash or any other specific symptoms and reports that, prior to this, the child was healthy. He has not had any recent illnesses, and, aside from some pediatric acetaminophen, has not taken any antibiotics or other medications. The child's birth history is unremarkable, with a vaginal delivery at 39 weeks, and the mother had all normal prenatal evaluations. According to the mother, the child has had normal growth, has received age-appropriate vaccinations, and has recently begun to walk and speak a few words. There are no smokers or sick contacts in the house, and there are no familial diseases. The child's diet has not changed, although he did recently visit family members in India for the first time. Currently, the mother is having trouble getting the child to eat food and drink the rehydration formula. The mother is extremely anxious and wants to know if her child needs to be admitted to the hospital.

Practice Case 29

Standardized Patient History-Taking Checklist

1.

2.

3.

4.

5.

6.

7.

8.

9.

10.

11.

12.

13.

14.

15.

16.

17.

HISTORY: Include significant positives and negatives from the history of present illness, past medical history, review of system(s), social history, and family history.

PHYSICAL EXAMINATION: Indicate only pertinent positive and negative findings related to the patient's chief complaint.

DIFFERENTIAL DIAGNOSIS

In order of likelihood (with 1 being most likely); list 5 possible diagnoses:

1.

2.

3.

4.

5.

DIAGNOSTIC WORKUP

List immediate plans (up to 5):

1.

2.

3.

4.

5.

PRACTICE CASE 30

Chart Information

Chief complaint: A 32-year-old woman comes to the clinic complaining of nipple discharge.

Vital signs: T: 37.1 C (98.8 F), BP: 122/72 mm Hg, HR: 84/min, RR: 14/min

History

About 2 weeks ago, the woman noticed a small amount of discharge from her left nipple. The discharge, which is "a few drops," has occurred most mornings since then, and it is often thin and clear or green tinged, although occasionally it will appear milky. The woman finally came to see you, as she saw what appeared to be bloody discharge 2 days ago. She is uncertain if there is a lump in her breast because she has had lumpy breasts since puberty, but she is concerned that there may well be one that is getting larger. There is no odor that the woman has noticed and she denies any fevers, pain, heat or cold intolerance, or similar symptoms in the past or in the other breast. There are no clear precipitating events or trauma, and nothing seems to improve or worsen her symptoms. Prior to this, she reports being healthy and has no significant medical conditions. She takes no medications and has no drug allergies. The woman reports that her mother died of ovarian cancer, her aunt died of breast cancer, and her father suffers from diabetes. Both her mother and aunt died in their forties. Her last menstrual period was 2 weeks ago. She is currently sexually active with her boyfriend and reports using condoms regularly. She does not smoke, drink, or use illicit substances.

Physical Examination

The patient appears comfortable and healthy. Inspection and palpation reveal no evidence of an enlarged thyroid gland. There are no palpable cervical, supraclavicular, or axillary lymph nodes. Chest is clear to auscultation bilaterally. Cardiovascular exam demonstrates normal sounds, rate and rhythm, without any murmurs, rubs, or gallops. On abdominal exam, percussion and palpation do not reveal an enlarged liver or spleen. She has normal active bowel sounds, and the abdomen is tympanic to percussion in all four quadrants. Her skin appears normal, without any obvious lesions.

Practice Case 30

Standardized Patient History-Taking Checklist

1.

2.

3.

4.

5.

6.

7.

8.

9.

10.

11.

12.

13.

14.

15.

16.

17.

18.

Standardized Patient Physical Examination Checklist

1.

2.

3.

4.

5.

6.

7.

8.

HISTORY: Include significant positives and negatives from the history of present illness, past medical history, review of system(s), social history, and family history.

PHYSICAL EXAMINATION: Indicate only pertinent positive and negative findings related to the patient's chief complaint.

DIFFERENTIAL DIAGNOSIS

In order of likelihood (with 1 being most likely); list 5 possible diagnoses:

1.

2.

3.

4.

5.

DIAGNOSTIC WORKUP

List immediate plans (up to 5):

1.

2.

3.

4.

5.

PRACTICE CASE 31

Chart Information

Chief complaint: A 54-year-old man complains of crying all the time.

Vital signs: T: 37 C (98.6 F), BP: 132/70 mm Hg, HR: 62/min, RR: 14/min

History

For the last year, the patient has suffered from a lack of energy and a severely depressed mood. He now finds himself crying daily for no particular reason and feels he does not have much to look forward to. There are few activities he still finds pleasurable. He no longer has much of an appetite and has difficulty staying asleep. He has alienated himself from friends and family and was recently fired after failing to show up to work on a regular basis. He is convinced this is proof that he is worthless. Additionally, he feels he is "wasting away" and has lost 15 lb over the past six months. He denies any other recent symptoms and specifically denies any heat or cold intolerance, constipation, or skin and hair changes. He cannot think of a precipitating event or anything that improves or worsens his symptoms. The patient has never suffered from such symptoms before and has never had any other psychiatric disturbances in the past. His past medical history is significant for a heart attack 1 year ago, high blood pressure, and rheumatoid arthritis. He has no known drug allergies and currently takes aspirin, atenolol, and prednisone. His family history is significant for heart disease and diabetes, but no psychiatric symptoms or disorders. He denies tobacco use but reports drinking a moderate amount. He states he did have a drug history in the past, but does not want to talk about it. Most days, the patient will have two to three "highballs," which he reports drinking both for his mood and his heart.

Physical/Mental Status Examination

The patient appears well groomed and alert and is in no obvious distress. He is alert and orient-ed to person, place, and time. His speech is mildly slow, but goal directed. He has no memory defects, either recent or remote. His attention and concentration are poor, as tested by serial sevens. His mood is depressed, and his affect is consistent. He does not have any hallucinations, delusions, or paranoias. He reports wishing "to end it all" but does not have a specific plan or time-line and has no desire to hurt others. He understands the severity of his condition, its impact on his life, and wants treatment. There is no evidence of an enlarged thyroid. His chest is clear to aus-cultation bilaterally. Cardiac examination reveals normal heart sounds, rate, and rhythm. There are no murmurs, rubs, or gallops. His extremities show no evidence of cyanosis, clubbing, edema. On abdominal exam, there is no evidence of hepatosplenomegaly, and the abdomen is tympanic in all four quadrants. He has normal active bowel sounds and is not tender on palpation. No abdominal masses are present.

Practice Case 31

Standardized Patient History-Taking Checklist

1.

2.

3.

4.

5.

6.

7.

8.

9.

10.

11.

12.

13.

14.

15.

16.

17.

Standardized Patient Physical Examination Checklist

1.

2.

3.

4.

5.

6.

7.

8.

9.

10.

11.

12.

13.

14.

15.

HISTORY: Include significant positives and negatives from the history of present illness, past medical history, review of system(s), social history, and family history.

PHYSICAL EXAMINATION: Indicate only pertinent positive and negative findings related to the patient's chief complaint.

DIFFERENTIAL DIAGNOSIS

In order of likelihood (with 1 being most likely); list 5 possible diagnoses:

1.

2.

3.

4.

5.

DIAGNOSTIC WORKUP

List immediate plans (up to 5):

1.

2.

3.

4.

5.

PRACTICE CASE 32

Chart Information

Chief complaint: A 52-year-old man complains of difficulty swallowing.

Vital signs: T: 37.3 C (99.1 F), BP: 148/78 mm Hg, HR: 74/min, RR: 16/min

History

For the last month, the patient has had progressive, constant difficulty swallowing food. At first, the man was able to compensate by chewing his food for longer than usual. However, his difficulty swallowing has progressed to the point that he has trouble with most meals. He cannot pinpoint a location where the problem is occurring, but it seems to be deep in his throat and occurs mainly after he has attempted to swallow some food. The problem, which he describes as severe, is only associated with solid food. He has no trouble with liquids or semisolid foods, such as applesauce or yogurt. He denies any severe pain associated with swallowing, but does sometimes have some mild (4/10) retrosternal pain. The pain is intermittent and seems to occur mostly at night. It does not spread to any other part of his body. He cannot think of anything that worsens or improves these symptoms. In addition to difficulty swallowing, he has noticed that he suffers from bad breath (which is unrelieved with breath mints), a 15-lb weight loss, and severe fatigue. He has also noticed some dark, foul-smelling stools and is now suffering from a hoarse voice, but otherwise reports feeling "okay." The patient denies any heat or cold intolerance, vomiting of blood, neck swelling, fevers, or skin and hair changes and doubts he swallowed anything he shouldn't have. He has never had any symptoms like this in the past and has generally been healthy. Past medical history is significant for hypertension, but aside from a daily aspirin, he takes no medications and has no known drug allergies. There are no similar symptoms or illnesses that run in his family. The patient denies smoking currently, having quit one year ago after a 30-year history of smoking 1 to 2 packs daily. He also denies drinking any alcohol over the past year, as he is a recovering alcoholic. He does not use any illicit drugs. He is not currently sexually active, though he reports a distant history of syphilis when he was in the Navy.

Physical Examination

The patient is tired and ill appearing. His throat shows no tonsillar enlargements, and there is no erythema or exudates. His mouth shows no evidence of lesions, vesicles, or thrush, and his dentition is good. His neck is supple, and thyroid appears and feels normal in size. There is no cervical, supraclavicular, or axillary lymphadenopathy. His chest is clear to auscultation bilaterally. Cardiovascular exam demonstrates normal sounds, rate and rhythm, without any murmurs, rubs, or gallops. The top of the jugular venous column appears at about 1 cm above the sternal notch. On abdominal exam, percussion and palpation do not reveal an enlarged liver or spleen. He has normal active bowel sounds, and the abdomen is tympanic to percussion in all four quadrants. There is no tenderness to palpation in any quadrant, and no masses are palpable.

Practice Case 32

Standardized Patient History-Taking Checklist

1.

2.

3.

4.

5.

6.

7.

8.

9.

10.

11.

12.

13.

14.

15.

16.

17.

Standardized Patient Physical Examination Checklist

1.

2.

3.

4.

5.

6.

7.

8.

9.

10.

11.

HISTORY: Include significant positives and negatives from the history of present illness, past medical history, review of system(s), social history, and family history.

PHYSICAL EXAMINATION: Indicate only pertinent positive and negative findings related to the patient's chief complaint.

DIFFERENTIAL DIAGNOSIS

In order of likelihood (with 1 being most likely); list 5 possible diagnoses:

1.

2.

3.

4.

5.

DIAGNOSTIC WORKUP

List immediate plans (up to 5):

1.

2.

3.

4.

5.

PRACTICE CASE 33

Chart Information

Chief complaint: A 33-year-old woman complains of hand swelling and stiffness.

Vital signs: T: 38.1 C (100.6 F), BP: 128/72 mm Hg, HR: 64/min, RR: 14/min

History

For the last 2 to 3 months, the patient reports symmetrical swelling and stiffness in both hands. The stiffness and a mild, dull, aching pain are of moderate (4/10) intensity and seem worse in the morning. The onset has been insidious, and the patient can think of no precipitating factors. She has noticed that the joints in her hands, particularly her knuckles, seem swollen when she first wakes up. By noon, the stiffness usually resolves. She has also had some soreness in her neck, lower back, and left knee, which feels similar. The woman has not noticed any rash or other skin lesions, swelling of her digits, visual changes, or urinary symptoms, but has had some low-grade fevers, significant, progressive fatigue, and an unintentional 10-lb weight loss. She has had facial rashes in the past, which she assumed to be acne. Over-the-counter pain medications, particularly ibuprofen and acetaminophen, have provided some relief, and she cannot think of anything in particular that has worsened her symptoms. She takes no other medications and has no drug allergies. Prior to this, she has never had any joint pain or similar events and has generally been healthy, although she did have one episode of chest pain diagnosed as pericarditis about 6 months ago. Her family history is remarkable only for psoriasis. She is currently sexually active with her husband of 5 years, uses an oral contraceptive pill, and has never had a sexually transmitted disease. There is no history of smoking, tobacco, or drug use. The woman works as a writer but has not been able to write more than a couple of paragraphs over the past two weeks, as her symptoms have been too severe.

Physical Examination

The woman is sitting comfortably on the examination table. Examination of her hands reveals no evidence of effusions, swelling of the digits, or warmth. She is able to flex and extend all of her joints without pain or stiffness. Her metacarpophalangeal joints and proximal interphalangeal joints are mildly tender to palpation. There are no swan-neck deformities, nodules, or swollen tendons. Her neck is supple and has a full range of motion without tenderness, as does her lower back. Her spinous processes reveal no abnormalities or tenderness to palpation and her knees exhibit no evidence of warmth or effusion. Chest is clear to auscultation bilaterally. Cardiovascular exam demonstrates normal sounds, rate and rhythm, without any murmurs, rubs, or gallops. On abdominal exam, percussion and palpation do not reveal an enlarged liver or spleen. She has normal active bowel sounds, and the abdomen is tympanic to percussion in all four quadrants. Her skin appears normal, without any obvious lesions.

Practice Case 33

Standardized Patient History-Taking Checklist

1.

2.

3.

4.

5.

6.

7.

8.

9.

10.

11.

12.

13.

14.

15.

16.

Standardized Patient Physical Examination Checklist

1.

2.

3.

4.

5.

6.

7.

8.

9.

10.

11.

12.

13.

HISTORY: Include significant positives and negatives from the history of present illness, past medical history, review of system(s), social history, and family history.

PHYSICAL EXAMINATION: Indicate only pertinent positive and negative findings related to the patient's chief complaint.

DIFFERENTIAL DIAGNOSIS

In order of likelihood (with 1 being most likely); list 5 possible diagnoses:

1.

2.

3.

4.

5.

DIAGNOSTIC WORKUP

List immediate plans (up to 5):

1.

2.

3.

4.

5.

PRACTICE CASE 34

Chart Information

Chief complaint: A 42-year-old woman comes to the emergency department with abdominal pain.

Vital signs: T: 38.8 C (101.8 F), BP: 120/72 mm Hg, HR: 98/min, RR: 14/min

History

The patient's pain began about 5 hours ago. It is located in the right upper quadrant of her abdomen and is severe, rating a 10/10 on a pain scale. The pain is dull and constant and started shortly after finishing dinner ("chicken fried steak," mashed potatoes, gravy, and peas). The pain seems to spread through to the upper part of her back and is associated with nausea and two episodes of greenish-yellow vomiting. Her pain is worse with deep inspiration and seems mildly improved by sitting upright. The woman denies any recent illnesses, fatigue, joint pain, abdominal pain in other locations, bloody or coffee-ground vomit, anorexia, or weight loss prior to her current symptoms. She has had episodes of dull, right upper quadrant pain, often after meals, but has never had pain this severe or long lasting. She takes no medications and has no drug allergies. Her past medical history is significant for pelvic inflammatory disease 2 years ago, multiple episodes of gonorrhea, an ectopic pregnancy, and alcoholism, although she has been sober for 3 years. She denies any changes in bowel frequency, consistency, or color. There is no significant family history; both parents and her brother are alive and healthy. The woman reports having three children, all of who are healthy. She is currently sexually active with two partners and states that she often uses condoms. There is no recent history of tobacco, alcohol, or drug use, although she did use intravenous heroin when she was in her twenties.

Physical Examination

The patient appears mildly uncomfortable and fidgety, although she is healthy appearing. The sclerae are normal. Her chest is clear to auscultation bilaterally, and tactile fremitus is within normal limits. Her cardiac exam demonstrates normal sounds, rate, and rhythm, without any murmurs, rubs, or peripheral edema. On abdominal exam, her liver and spleen are not enlarged, although her abdomen is obese. She has normal active bowel sounds, and her abdomen is tympanic to percussion in all four quadrants. She is tender to palpation in the right upper quadrant of her abdomen, but displays no rebound tenderness or guarding. She has a positive Murphy sign. She has no costovertebral angle or flank tenderness. Her skin appears normal, without discoloration or rash.

Practice Case 34

Standardized Patient History-Taking Checklist

1.

2.

3.

4.

5.

6.

7.

8.

9.

10.

11.

12.

13.

14.

15.

Standardized Patient Physical Examination Checklist

1.

2.

3.

4.

5.

6.

7.

8.

9.

10.

HISTORY: Include significant positives and negatives from the history of present illness, past medical history, review of system(s), social history, and family history.

PHYSICAL EXAMINATION: Indicate only pertinent positive and negative findings related to the patient's chief complaint.

DIFFERENTIAL DIAGNOSIS

In order of likelihood (with 1 being most likely); list 5 possible diagnoses:

1.

2.

3.

4.

5.

DIAGNOSTIC WORKUP

List immediate plans (up to 5):

1.

2.

3.

4.

5.

PRACTICE CASE 35

Chart Information

Chief complaint: A 52-year-old man comes to the emergency department with shortness of breath.

Vital signs: T: 37 C (98.6 F), BP: 102/68 mm Hg, HR: 96/min, RR: 24/min

History

For the last 2 to 3 months, the patient has had repeated episodes of shortness of breath. This sensation usually occurs with exertion and has been getting progressively worse. Now the man has trouble climbing stairs without becoming fatigued. He estimates he can walk less than one city block before becoming extremely short of breath. Over the last two weeks, he has had a mild cough, occasionally productive of pink-tinged, thin, frothy sputum, and a subjective low-grade fever. His symptoms are worse when he lies down, and he has recently had to sleep in a recliner. When he tries to sleep flat, he will occasionally awake gasping for air, although his symptoms improve when he sits upright. Additionally, he has significant swelling in his legs and a 10-lb weight gain over the last month, despite having no appetite. He denies any recent chest pain, shaking chills, wheeze, muscle or joint aches, or urinary symptoms, although he is getting up frequently throughout the night to use the bathroom. He has had not had any episodes of nausea, vomiting, or sweating. The only thing that has helped his symptoms is some furosemide that he borrowed from his wife. He can think of no precipitating events. Since taking this medication, his swelling has resolved and his cough and shortness of breath have improved. In addition to this medication, he takes a baby aspirin, metoprolol, and simvastatin. He has had similar symptoms once before, about 2 years ago, when he was hospitalized for a myocardial infarction. His medical history is also significant for high blood pressure and hyperlipidemia. The patient has no known drug allergies. Family history is significant for a brother and father who died of myocardial infarctions in their forties. The man currently smokes about half-a-pack a day and has done so for 30 years, although he is trying to quit. He denies alcohol or drug use.

Physical Examination

The patient appears comfortable and in no distress. He appears to be breathing at a rate of approximately 20 to 25 breaths/min, and he coughs when asked to breathe deeply or expire fully. He is not using any accessory muscles of respiration, and his chest wall appears symmetrical. Rales are heard at lung bases bilaterally, and tactile fremitus is normal. There is 2+ pitting edema of the lower extremities. His heart demonstrates normal sounds, rate, and rhythm. There are no murmurs, rubs, or gallops present. The point of maximal impulse is not displaced and is of normal size. The top of his jugular venous fluid column appears at approximately 2 cm above his sternoclavicular notch. On abdominal exam, the liver is not enlarged. He has normal active bowel sounds, and the abdomen is tympanic to percussion in all four quadrants with no tenderness on palpation.

Practice Case 35

Standardized Patient History-Taking Checklist

1.

2.

3.

4.

5.

6.

7.

8.

9.

10.

11.

12.

13.

14.

Standardized Patient Physical Examination Checklist

1.

2.

3.

4.

5.

6.

7.

8.

9.

10.

HISTORY: Include significant positives and negatives from the history of present illness, past medical history, review of system(s), social history, and family history.

PHYSICAL EXAMINATION: Indicate only pertinent positive and negative findings related to the patient's chief complaint.

DIFFERENTIAL DIAGNOSIS

In order of likelihood (with 1 being most likely); list 5 possible diagnoses:

1.

2.

3.

4.

5.

DIAGNOSTIC WORKUP

List immediate plans (up to 5):

1.

2.

3.

4.

5.

| SECTION TWO |

Appendices

Appendix I: **Abbreviations**

Use abbreviations sparingly. For clarity, it is always better to spell out the acronym or abbreviation.

yo	year old
m	male
f	female
b	black
w	white
L	left
R	right
hx	history
h/o	history of
c/o	complaining/complaints of
NL	normal limits
WNL	within normal limits
Ø	without or no
+	positive
–	negative
abd	abdomen
AIDS	acquired immune deficiency syndrome
AP	anteroposterior
BUN	blood urea nitrogen
CABG	coronary artery bypass grafting
CBC	complete blood count
CCU	cardiac care unit
cig	cigarettes
CHF	congestive heart failure
COPD	chronic obstructive pulmonary disease
CPR	cardiopulmonary resuscitation
CT	computed tomography
CVA	cerebrovascular accident
CVP	central venous pressure
CXR	chest x-ray
DM	diabetes mellitus
DTR	deep tendon reflexes

ECG	electrocardiogram
ED	emergency department
EMT	emergency medical technician
ENT	ears, nose, and throat
EOM	extraocular muscles
ETOH	alcohol
Ext	extremities
FH	family history
GI	gastrointestinal
GU	genitourinary
HEENT	head, eyes, ears, nose, and throat
HIV	human immunodeficiency virus
HPI	history of present illness
HTN	hypertension
IM	intramuscularly
IV	intravenously
JVD	kidney, ureter, and bladder
LMP	last menstrual period
LP	lumbar puncture
MI	myocardial infarction
MRI	magnetic resonance imaging
MVA	motor vehicle accident
Neuro	neurologic
NIDDM	non–insulin-dependent diabetes mellitus
NKA	no known allergies
NKDA	no known drug allergy
NSR	normal sinus rhythm
PA	posteroanterior
PERLA	pupils are equal and reactive to light and accommodation
po	orally
PT	prothrombin time
PTT	partial prothrombin time
RBC	red blood cells
SH	social history
TIA	transient ischemic attack
U/A	urinalysis
URI	upper respiratory tract infection
WBC	white blood cells

Appendix II: **Step 2 CS In a Nutshell**

THE DIFFERENTIAL DIAGNOSIS

Each standardized patient (SP) encounter will require you to exhibit your ability in data gathering. This part of the Step 2 CS is accomplished through the taking of a patient history and conducting an appropriate physical examination. During this time, the questions you ask and the maneuvers you do are meant to help you narrow the possible conditions or illnesses that the SP may have. This is called establishing a differential diagnosis.

The differential diagnosis process actually begins *outside* the examination room with the posted patient information. This information contains the patient's age, chief complaint or reason for this visit, and location of the encounter, e.g., a 58-year-old man presents to the clinic with chest pain of several hours' duration. This "doorway information" sets the stage for the encounter by enabling you to come up with a *mental list* of possible *common* diagnoses before the actual encounter starts. For instance, in this case of a 58-year-old man with chest pain of several hours' duration, the possible causes of his chest pain are not unlimited, but there are still a great number of possible causes. Some common causes of chest pain in a man of this age include: *1*) MI, *2*) angina, *3*) pneumonia, *4*) GERD, and *5*) costochondritis. Remember also to consider the patient's vital signs before you enter the room. They may cause you to immediately reprioritize your list. For example, in this case, if the patient presented with fever, you might consider adjusting your mental list to: *1*) pneumonia, *2*) MI, *3*) angina, *4*) GERD, or *5*) costochondritis.

Once *inside* the examination room, your history should pursue a line of questioning mindful of the diagnoses you are considering from the doorway information. Use your initial doorway considerations as a guide, but be careful. Your questioning may lead you to adjust the priority of the diagnoses you are considering, add other possibilities not yet considered as part of your mental list, or even pare down your differential list to only one or two possibilities. Obviously, the questions you ask should attempt to eliminate as many options in the fewest number of questions, while retaining those that could be the most likely causes. Based on the presenting problem(s), you'll likely ask a series of questions meant to narrow the possible cause(s) of the problem to the most likely ones. Make sure to use open-ended questions, facilitation, clarification, and repetition to help analyze the patient's condition. As you do the history, return to the chief complaint when necessary to make sure that you are still following the correct diagnostic path. Once you have completed the history, while washing your hands, reprioritize your diagnoses based on all the information attained to this point. From this analysis you will plan out what to include in your physical examination.

Next, perform the physical exam on those systems you are strongly considering for the differential diagnosis, in the order that you are considering them. Thus, in this case, if after the history you are still considering the same differentials in the same order, i.e., *1*) pneumonia, *2*) MI, *3*) angina, *4*) GERD, *5*) costochondritis, then examine the lungs first, followed by the heart, the sternum, and then the abdomen. The rationale here is that time will be limited, and you want to make sure you have at least examined those systems that are most likely to be involved. Keep in mind that during the physical you may need to continue asking questions, though these would be mostly related to the exam itself (e.g., "Does it hurt when I press here?"). However, additional questions about the history may also need to be asked during the physical as you narrow down and reprioritize the differentials. Following the physical, make one final adjustment to your mental differential list and develop a plan for further studies to pinpoint the patient's actual diagnosis.

Common Errors in the Differential Diagnosis Process

Determining the proper differential diagnosis is one of the keys to passing the Step 2 CS. Asking the wrong questions leads to mistakes in the differential diagnosis, which then leads to performing the incorrect physical exam, resulting in a failing score on the data gathering section of the Step 2 CS.

In general, there are four common errors that can occur when doing the differential diagnosis.

1. Skipping steps in the data-gathering process

This usually occurs when taking the patient history. It is easy to fixate on one piece of information from the initial answers and then follow a line of questioning that fails to elicit other pertinent information. And because the history is the single most important source of information used in arriving at the differential diagnosis, jumping to conclusions can lead to an incorrect differential.

Solution

1. Keep a list in your mind of all the common possible differential diagnoses, and adjust it as necessary throughout the case.

2. Ask questions that positively eliminate or reprioritize possible differentials.

3. Check with the patient that there are no other symptoms that may lead to other diagnoses. ("So, you have had a cough for the past week and a fever. Are there any other problems that you have had?")

4. Listen closely to the patient's answers, and don't cut him or her off by immediately asking another question or appearing to be ready to ask another question.

2. Using the wrong information

Even when you have asked the right questions and feel that you have eliminated possible choices in the differential diagnosis for the right reasons, it is still possible to use the wrong information in making your decisions. For example, in response to your question, "Do you smoke?" the patient says, "No." But had you asked, "Do you use tobacco?," the patient's answer might have been, "I don't smoke, but I do chew."

Solution

1. Clarify the answers that the patient gives you to be sure that you correctly understand what they mean. ("You said that you have never smoked. Have you used any other tobacco product, like snuff or chew?")

2. Ask yourself whether an answer can be complete or accurate, given the patient's age, sex, or other history. ("You said that both your parents, your siblings, and your wife all smoke, but that you don't. Have you ever used any other tobacco product, like snuff or chew?")

3. Restricting or limiting the problem

It is incorrect to limit or restrict your differential diagnosis based on your own preconceived assumptions of the patient's conditions. Doing so will prematurely bring closure to a line of questioning that may in fact be valid. For example, a patient comes in whom you suspect is a drug addict because of the way he is dressed and his physical mannerisms (licking lips, runny nose, bloodshot eyes, dirty). Because of this misconception, you fail to ask questions about the patient's history that would identify him as suffering from pneumonia, and you fail to believe him when he says that he is not a drug addict.

Solution

1. Perform the workup based on the information given. Don't make any assumptions or jump to conclusions.

2. Be objective in your assessment of the patient's condition. Don't let physical appearances (either positive or negative) influence your rapport with the patient.

4. Giving up on a problem too soon

This usually means giving up on a patient too soon. Because of memory, language (i.e., poor vocabulary, accent), or emotional problems (e.g., anxiety, anger), which can make communicating with the patient difficult, it is often easier to cut short the interview and progress straight to the physical examination.

Solution

1. Facilitate communication by encouraging the patient to explain the problem in his or her own words. Repeat or paraphrase what is said to make sure you understand completely.

2. Remember, the patient is the best source of information about his or her condition. There is no real substitute for what patient knows and no better way to determine the problem than to ask directly.

3. Most importantly, show that you care and are concerned about the patient's health with verbal and physical reassurances.

Appendix III: **Step-by-Step Through a General SP History**

Ask the Patient for the Chief Complaint

To begin the patient encounter, greet the patient (smiling): "Ms. Smith, hello. Let me introduce myself. My name is Dr. Reina. I'm a doctor here in the hospital. It is nice to meet you. I would like to ask you a few questions and do a physical exam. So let's get started."

- What caused you to come in today?

    or

    What made you come in today?

    What made you want to see a doctor today?

    What caused you to come into the clinic today?

    What problem brought you in today?

History of Present Illness

Progression of symptoms from beginning to present

- **When** did this first begin? *or* When did this problem start? *or* How long have you had this?
- **Have** you ever had anything like this before?

Questions addressing common symptoms

- How would you **describe** the pain (feeling, discomfort)?

    or

    Please describe how it feels.

    Tell me what it feels like.

If patient needs prompting:

Is it a dull ache (sharp, stabbing, burning, pulling, pulsating, cramping, pressure)?

Does it come and go?

Is the pain there all the time?

- If 10 is the worst pain you've ever had, **where is this on a scale of 1 to 10?**

KAPLAN **medical**

- Where is the pain **located**?

     or

  Please show me exactly where the pain is.

  Can you show me where it hurts?

  Exactly where is the pain?

  Can you point to the place where you're hurting?

  With one finger, please touch the spot where you feel the pain.

  Where is the pain (discomfort)?

- Does the pain **move** anywhere? Show me where. (Note: Don't use the word "radiate.")

     or

  Do you feel the pain anywhere else?

  Does it ever travel to any other part of your body?

  Does this pain ever move around?

- How **often** do you have this? *or* When do you get these pains (feelings)? *or* When does this occur?

- Are you aware of anything that might have **brought this on**?

     or

  What happened right before this came on (started)?

  What happened at that time?

  Did anything unusual happen at that time?

  Was anything unusual happening when this first started?

  About the time that this problem began, was there any special event that occurred?

- Does anything make your pain **worse**?

     or

  Does anything make it worse?

  What makes it worse?

  Does anything make you feel worse?

- Does anything make your pain **better**?

     or

  Does anything make it better?

  What makes it better?

  Does anything make you feel better?

- In addition to your headache, have you noticed anything else (e.g., nausea, vomiting, cough, fever, dizziness, cold, sore throat, weakness in your legs, tingling sensation, burning sensation, numbness, sweating)?

- Did or do you feel **nauseated**?

  or

  Have you been nauseated?

  Did you feel sick to your stomach?

- Did you **vomit?**

  or

  Did you throw up?

  Have you been vomiting?

  and

  What was in it?

  What **color** was it?

  Was there any **blood** in it?

  How **much** was there?

- When you **cough**, does anything come up?

  or

  Do you ever spit (cough) anything up?

  and

  What **color** is it?

  Is there any **blood** in it?

  How **much** phlegm comes up?

- Have you been having **headaches**?

  or

  Do you get headaches?

  and

  Where are your headaches?

  How **intense** (painful) are they on a scale from 1 to 10 (10 being the worst)?

  When did they start?

  How often do you get a headache?

  What are you doing when the headache comes on?

- Have you been running a **fever**?

  or

  Have you been feeling hotter (warmer) than usual?

  and

  Do you **sweat** a lot during the **night**?

- Do you get **short of breath**?

  or

  Do you ever feel out of breath?

  and

  Have you been **wheezing**?

- Have you had any changes in your **urinary** habits?

- Have you had any changes in your **bowel** habits?

    and

    When you go to the bathroom, what does your stool look like?

    What color is it?

    Was it very foul smelling?

    Does it float?

    Have you been having diarrhea?

    How long have you had the diarrhea?

    Have you been constipated?

    How many bowel movements do you have per day?

    Do you get stomach cramps?

- Has your **weight changed** any?

    and

    Over what period of time?

- Have your **eating habits changed** in any way?

    or

    What do you usually eat?

    Did you eat anything unusual?

    What did you eat right before the nausea started?

- Has your sleep pattern changed in any way?
- Have there been any changes in your **vision**?

    or

    Has your eyesight changed in any way?

- Do you ever feel **dizzy**?

    or

    Do you have blackout sensations?

- Do you have **joint pain** anywhere in your body?

    or

    Do you have pain in any other joints?

- Have there been any changes in your **environment** lately?

- Have you been **traveling** anywhere lately?

Past medical history (make sure to specify any pertinent "yes" or "no" answers)

- Have you ever had this or a **similar experience** before?
- Have you ever had _____? Name diseases or conditions related to chief complaint and history findings.
- Have you ever had to stay in the **hospital** overnight?
- Have you ever had **surgery**?
- Have you had any recent **injuries or accidents**?
- Are you taking any **medications**? Ask about prescriptions, over-the-counter meds, vitamins, or herbs.
- Do you have any **allergies** (strange reactions), such as to medications, foods, animals, or plants?

Family history

- Does anyone in your family have this or a **similar problem**?
- Then ask about specific related illnesses or conditions.
- Then ask, "In addition to that, are there any serious illnesses or conditions in your family?"

Sexual history

- Are you currently **sexually active**? (If yes, do you use condoms consistently? Other contraceptives?)
- How many sexual partners have you had over the past 6 months?
- Have you ever had a **sexually transmitted disease**?
- Have you ever been tested for HIV?
- Are your sexual partners men, women, or both?
- Do you have any problems with sexual function? (or with having erections?)

Social history

- Have you ever used tobacco in any form? (If yes, how many packs for smoking a day and for how many years?)
- Do you **drink alcohol**? (If yes, how much and how often?)
- Do you use any **recreational drugs**? (If yes, which ones? How often? Do you inject any drugs?)
- Tell me about your work situation. Is there physical strain? Are you exposed to hazardous materials? Is it stressful?

    and

- Tell me about your home life.

Gynecologic/obstetric history

- How old were you when you had your first period?
- Do you have a period every month?
- When was your last menstrual period?
- How many days are in your cycle?
- Has your period changed in any way?
- Do you have cramps?

• On a heavy day, how many pads or tampons do you use?

• Do you ever have any spotting (breakthrough bleeding) between periods?

• Do you have any problems with PMS?

• Have you ever been pregnant? (If yes, how many times? How many children have you had?)

• Have you ever had a miscarriage or abortion? (If miscarried, in what trimester?)

Taking a Pediatric History

• No children present

• Anxious parents (use good communication skills)

• Can order physical exam for child

• What to ask:

  – Obtain HPI just as in adults
  – Birth history, prenatal history
  – Growth/Development history
  – Immunizations
  – Family history
  – Past medical history
  – Allergies
  – Smokers in the home?
  – Meds

• Case to expect–sick child at home or failure to thrive

TAKING A PEDIATRIC HISTORY

Birth History

• Was the pregnancy full term? (40 weeks or 9 months)

• Did the mother have routine prenatal checkups? How often?

• Was a sonogram or amniocentesis performed during the pregnancy?

• Were there any problems with the pregnancy?

• Did the mother smoke, drink, or use drugs during the pregnancy?

• Was it a normal, uncomplicated, vaginal delivery?

• Did the child have any medical problems when he or she was born?

• Mother and child left the hospital after how long?

Feeding History

• Was the child breastfed or given formula?

• Started eating solid food when?

• Eats and likes what foods now?

• How is the child's appetite?

• Does the child take a daily pediatric multiple vitamin?

• Does the child have any allergies?

Routine Care

• Name of pediatrician and clinic where child is routinely seen?

• Up-to-date immunizations? (hepatitis B, DPT, and polio "series shots"; MMR)

• Date of child's last routine checkup?

• Has the child ever been hospitalized?

• Any serious illnesses?

• Any medications?

TAKING A PSYCHIATRIC HISTORY

Special Aspects

- Past psychiatric history
- Med/drugs/ETOH
- Family psychiatric history
- Social history
- Psychiatric mental status
  - Appearance
  - Consciousness
  - Orientation
  - Speech
  - Memory
  - Attention/concentration
  - Mood
  - Affect
  - Perceptions
  - Suicidal/homicidal ideation
  - Judgment/insight

Psychiatric Questions

Source of unhappiness (anxiety, frustration, feelings, mood change)

- Do you have any idea of what is causing your unhappiness (sadness, confusion)?
- Would you be willing to share with me what happened that made you feel this way?

Support systems

- Do you have anyone you can talk to?
- Do you have any friends or family members you relate to?
- Is there anyone there for you when you need them?

Appetite

- Has your appetite changed any?
- Do you feel like eating?
- Have your eating habits changed any?

Weight

- Has your weight changed any?

Caffeine

- How's your caffeine intake?
- Do you have a lot of coffee, colas, tea, or chocolate?

Note

When taking a psychiatric history, ask more open-ended questions than usual (e.g., "Tell me more about that."; "What has this been like for you?").

Daily routine

- Has your daily routine changed any?
- What do you usually do with your time?

Sleep pattern

- Is your sleep affected by this?
- Have your sleeping patterns (habits) changed in any way?

Interests/activities

- What kind of interests/activities do you have?
- What activities are you involved in?
- Have your interests/activities changed at all?
- Do you feel any pleasure from the things you're involved in?

Concentration/memory

- How's your concentration (memory)?
- Are you having any difficulty concentrating (remembering things)?
- Do you lose things more often?

Duration of affect

- How long have you been feeling this way?

Optimism/pessimism

- Do you have any plans for the future?
- What are your plans for the future?
- Would you say you usually feel optimistic or pessimistic?
- Do you think things will get any better?

Ideation of suicide or self-inflicted pain

- Do you ever consider taking your own life?
- Do you ever imagine ending your life?
- Do you ever think about killing yourself?
- Do you ever feel like ending it all?
- Do you ever feel tempted to take your life?
- Do you think you might want to kill yourself?

Suicidal plan

- Do you actually have a plan?
- Would you be willing to tell me what it is?
- Do you already have the gun (pills)?

Abuse

- Are you in any danger from anyone in your personal life?
- Tell me about your home life.
- Do you feel safe at home (in your relationships)?
- Do your parents (boyfriend/girlfriend, roommate, husband/wife) treat you badly, i.e., How's your relationship with your parents?
- You're wearing an ace bandage on your wrist. Can you tell me about that?
- Were you harmed repeatedly by anyone during your childhood?
- Were you left alone often?
- Does anyone repeatedly call you names or put you down?

Harming others

- Do you ever feel like hurting anyone?

Hallucinations

- Sometimes when people are under a lot of stress, they see or hear things that others don't. Does this ever happen to you?
- Do people ever tell you they think you're hearing or seeing things that others don't?

Delusions

- Do people ever say they think you have extremely unrealistic ideas about yourself or about life in general?

Mini-mental status

If you notice that the patient seems to be hearing "voices" or seeing things during the encounter; if you get positive responses to questions about hallucination, delusion, and concentration/ memory impairment; or if the patient seems to be unusually confused or distant, you may want to invest some of your time in doing a part of the mental status exam. Don't spend too much time on it, and don't just lunge right into it. Introduce it by saying: "I'd like to check your memory and concentration by asking you to do a few things now." When doing this, you can also check their orientation, speech, attention, mood, affect, and perceptions (hallucinations, paranoias, suicidal/homicidal ideation, judgment, insight).

Thyroid function

- Do you often get constipated?
- Has your skin been really dry lately?
- Have you been losing your hair? (Has your hair been falling out?)
- Do cold or hot temperatures ever bother you very badly?
- Do you have trouble sleeping?

Family history

- Has anyone in your family ever had problems with feeling low or extremely discouraged in life?
- Does anyone in your family have problems with concentration or clear thinking?

Note

Documentation of the Mental Status Exam

Mental status: Patient appears well groomed/unkempt.

He/she is alert/stuporous/lethargic and oriented/disoriented to person, place, time.

Speech is fluid/pressured/slow and goal directed/tangential.

Recent and remote memory are/are not intact.

Attention and concentration are good/impaired as tested by serial sevens.

Mood is euthymic/depressed/ euphoric. Affect is/is not consistent with mood.

The patient does/does not have abnormal hallucinations, delusion, paranoias.

The patient denies/admits having suicidal/homicidal ideation or intent.

Judgment/insight are intact/impaired.

Willingness to seek help

- Would you like to talk things over with a counselor?
- Would you be willing to let a counselor help you work through this problem?
- There are several good support groups in the community. Would you like to have this kind of peer support?
- A good counselor can help you through this difficult time. Would you like a list of professionals in the local area?
- I just want you to know you're not alone. There are people ready to help you make it through this. I can get a list of phone numbers you can call if you need help.

Psych Differentials

- Adjustment disorder
- Drug/alcohol use
- Med side effects
- Delirium
- Dementia
- Acute confusional state
- Brief psychotic reaction
- Bipolar disorder
- Unipolar major depression
- Underlying medical disorder
    - SLE
    - HIV
    - Pheochromocytoma
    - Thyroid
    - DM
    - Infection
    - Brain tumor

Psych Tests

- CT or MRI brain
- TSH, T_3, T_4
- Drug screen
- Electrolytes
- Urine for catecholamines, VMA
- HIV ELISA
- Vitamin B_{12}, folate, RPR

KAPLAN
medical

MINI MENTAL STATUS EXAM

/ / Alzheimer dementia
/ / Multi-infarct dementia
/ / Mixed dementias
/ / Other _____

Score		
	Orientation	
( )	What is the (year) (season) (month) (date) (day)?	(5 points)
( )	Where are we? (state) (country) (town) (hospital) (floor)	(5 points)
	Registration	
( )	Name 3 objects: 1 second to say each. Then ask the patient to repeat all 3 after you have said them. 1 point for each correct. Then repeat them until s/he learns them. Count trials and record. _____	(3 points)
	Attention and Calculation	
( )	Serial 7s: 1 point for each correct. Stop at 5 answers. Or spell "world" backwards. (Number correct equals letters before the first mistake, i.e., "d-l-o-r-w" = 2 correct.)	(5 points)
	Recall	
( )	Ask for the objects above. 1 point for each correct.	(3 points)
	Language Tests	
( )	Name: pencil, watch	(2 points)
( )	Repeat: "no ifs, ands, or buts"	(1 point)
( )	Follow a three-stage command: "Take the paper in your hand, fold it in half, and put it on the floor."	(3 points)
	Read and Obey the Following:	
( )	Close your eyes.	(1 point)
( )	Write a sentence spontaneously below.	(1 point)
( )	Copy design below.	(1 point)

( )	Total (30 points)	

KAPLAN
medical

FUNCTIONAL STATUS EXAM

Functioning

Activities of Daily Living—involves basic activities

- Feeding (as long as you don't have to use appliances)
- Bathing (sponge baths; doesn't include operating complex shower knobs)
- Toileting
- Dressing (not considering color matches, appropriateness, etc.)
- Ambulating
- Transferring from bed
- Transferring from toilet
- Bowel and bladder control
- Grooming (not including use of electric razor or electric toothbrush)

Instrumental Activities of Daily Living—involves use of machines/instruments

- Cooking
- Cleaning
- Using telephone (making call, not receiving)
- Writing
- Shopping* (considered a high-level "executive" activity)
- Laundry
- Managing medication (selecting, sorting, taking on time)
- Using public transportation*
- Walking outdoors without getting lost*
- Managing money (paying bills and maintaining bankbook)
- Traveling out of town by oneself*
- Driving*

Reasoning

Abstract—tested with use of proverbs

- Patients who have difficulty with abstract reasoning explain proverbs concretely. For example, ask the patient what "people who live in houses shouldn't throw stones" means. A concrete answer would be something like, "If you throw a stone, you might break the glass."
- "The early bird catches the worm" is another proverb. A concrete answer might be along the lines of: "If a bird gets up early in the morning to look for food, he is more likely to find a worm."
- Other proverbs include: "don't count your chickens before they are hatched"; "a stitch in time saves nine"; "the restless sleeper blames the couch"; "a rolling stone gathers no moss"; and "the mouse that has but one hole is soon caught."
- Another way to test reasoning is to ask the patient to explain similarities and/or differences between such things as an orange and an apple, a cat and a mouse, or a church and a theatre.

---

*Not appropriate for homebound patients.

Orientation

- **Person**—Ask the person his name. If you ask him who you are, he might know he is talking to a doctor but may not remember your name unless you are wearing a nametag.
- **Place**—Ask the patient to name the place where your interaction is occurring. He might say that it is a large building or even a hospital, but he may not be able to name the hospital.
- **Time**—This includes the season, year, month, date, and day of the week. With mild impairment, the patient may know the season and month but may be confused with the day of the week, the month, or the year.

Memory

- **Immediate**—To test immediate memory, see if the patient can immediately repeat the names of three objects or three numbers.
- **Short-term**—Ask the patient to repeat the same three objects or numbers after 5 minutes have elapsed.
- **Recent**—Ask the patient about a news event that was reported, what he watched on TV last night, or what the weather was like yesterday. Ask for information that can be verified.

Attention/Concentration

- Subtracting serial sevens is a difficult test because it involves attention and concentration. Ask the patient to start from 100 and subtract by sevens. This test is only valid if the patient has had at least a fourth-grade education. If serial sevens seems impaired, the patient may still be able to count by twos, fives, or tens because that is done by rote.
- A similar test is asking the patient to spell a simple word forward and backward. A word that is commonly used for this is "world".

Judgment

Judgment can be tested by giving the patient a situation to resolve. Ask the patient, "What would you do if you found a stamped and addressed envelope?" or "What would you do if you saw smoke in the wastepaper basket?" or "What would you do if you needed medical attention?"

Emotional State

Describe your impression of the patient's emotional state. This can be assessed by your interactions with the patient throughout the encounter. Use adjectives such as "normal," "depressed," "hostile," etc. (Use segments from the mini-mental status exam if you suspect problems.)

Intellect

- Intellect is usually assessed by your interactions with the patient throughout the encounter. However, if you suspect problems, then test for this by asking specific questions.
- **Fund of knowledge**—Ask questions that are consistent with the patient's level of education and background.

KAPLAN
medical

Use of Language

- **Name objects.** Ask the patient to name simple objects, such as a pen, safety pin, chair, etc.

- **Follow commands.** This is usually tested by giving the patient one, two, or three commands at the same time. A patient with impairment may be able to follow one or two commands but may have trouble with three. An example might be to take a piece of paper, fold it in half, and place it on the floor.

- **Speech evaluation.** This is done incidentally throughout the encounter. If you suspect problems, see specifics in the mini mental status exam.

- **Right/left orientation.** Ask the patient to do something with his right or left hand. The patient may confuse right and left but still know which hand he writes with.

- **Writing/visual spatial ability.** Ask the patient to write a complete sentence of his choice (do not dictate the sentence). See if the patient stays on the line and maintains a constant letter size. The sentence should contain a subject and a verb. You can also ask the patient to copy a simple picture, such as interlocking pentagons.

- **Drawing ability.** Ask the patient to draw the face of a clock to judge his perception and construction of the object. Check for spatial distortion and numerical order. The hands of the clock should also be in direct proportion to the face.

Appendix IV: **Suggested Phrasing of Instructions for the Physical Exam**

The next several pages contain suggested phrasing for each system of the physical exam. Please note that some may seem obvious, whereas others do not. Please extract the information that is most relevant to your comfort and experience level.

Table IV-1. HEENT Examination

Action	Suggested Phrasing	Comments
Palpation of head	"I need to press lightly on your head."	
Palpation of sinuses	"Now let me press lightly on your face."	
Palpation of ears	"Now I'll press around your ears. I need to pull up on your ears now."	
Palpation of lymph nodes	"I need to check your neck for swollen glands."	"Lymph nodes" is medical terminology.
Otoscope Eyes Nose Throat	"Please pick a point on the wall and look at it. I'm going to check your eyes." "I'm going to check your nose." "Please stick your tongue out and say 'ah'. Thank you."	
Weber	"Now I need to check your hearing. I'm going to put this tuning fork on your head. Tell me if it sounds the same in both ears."	
Rinne	"I'm going to put the tuning fork behind your ear. Tell me when you can't hear it any longer. Can you hear it now?"	
Thyroid Auscultation of gland Palpation of gland	"Now I need to check your neck area." "I'm going to press lightly on your neck, so I'll need you to swallow. Would you like some water? Okay, let me get it. Please take a drink and hold it until I ask you to swallow."	The word "thyroid" may be considered medical terminology. Demonstrates empathy to offer water to help patient swallow more easily. If patient doesn't want water, don't insist.
Palpation of skin	"I need to check your skin."	
Hair brittleness	"I need to check your hair."	
Check for tremors	"Please hold our your hands like this and close your eyes."	Demonstrate how patient should hold hands.

KAPLAN
medical

Table IV-2. Neurologic Examination

Action	Suggested Phrasing	Comments
PERRLA	"I need to check your eyes."	
Funduscopic	"Now I need to shine the light so I can examine the back of your eyes. Thank you."	If patient resists, say, "I need to look at the blood vessels back there to make sure they're not damaged. It's extremely important for your safety."
Cranials 3, 4, 6 5 5 7 7 9, 10 11 12	"Please follow my finger without moving your head." "Please clench your jaws." "I'm going to touch your face lightly. Do you feel this? Now please close your eyes. Do you feel this? How about this? Is it the same?" "Please raise your eyebrows." "Please smile and show me your teeth." "Please stick out your tongue and say, 'ah'." "Now shrug your shoulders." "Now please stick out your tongue and move it from side to side."	Do for all three branches. Afterward, say, "Now you may open your eyes." If any sentence is difficult for you to pronounce, just demonstrate the action and say, "Do this."
Upper extremities Muscle testing Reflexes Sensory Light touch Sharp and dull	"Now I'll check your arm strength. Do this. Don't let me push in. Don't let me push out. Do this. Don't let me push up. Don't let me push down. Do this. Don't let me squeeze your fingers together. Do this. Squeeze my fingers as hard as you can." "Now I need to tap on your arms." "Now I need to check your sense of touch." "Now I'm going to touch your hands lightly. Tell me if you feel it. Does it feel the same? Okay, now close your eyes." "Now I need to check your sharp and dull sensation. This is sharp. This is dull. Please close your eyes and tell me what you feel. Which is this? And this? How about this?"	Remember "MRS": <u>M</u>uscles <u>R</u>eflexes <u>S</u>ensation Repeat for three points on hand. Afterward, say, "Okay, you may open your eyes now." Repeat for three points on hand. Then say, "Please open your eyes."

(Continued)

KAPLAN
medical

Table IV-2. Neurologic Examination (*continued*)

Action	Suggested Phrasing	Comments
Lower extremities	"I need to check your leg strength. May I raise the sheet? Thank you."	
Muscle testing	"Push out. Pull back. Push on the gas [or] Push down. Pull up."	
Reflexes	"Now I'm going to tap on your legs."	Tap in two areas.
Babinski	"Now I need to tickle (or scratch) your feet lightly."	
Sensory		
Light touch	"I'm going to touch your legs lightly. Tell me if you feel this. Please close your eyes. Do you feel this? This? Does it feel the same?"	Repeat for four points. Then say, "Please open your eyes."
Sharp and dull	"Now I need to check your responses to sharp and dull touch. This is sharp. This is dull. Please close your eyes. Which is this? How about this?"	Repeat for four points on feet. Then say, "Please open your eyes."
Cerebellar		
Finger to nose	"Please touch your nose with this finger, then touch mine."	Be sure to hold up your own index finger to demonstrate.
Heel to shin	"Please do this. Do the same with your other leg."	
Gait	"Now I need to see how you walk. Let me pull out the footstool. May I help you step down? Please walk to the other side of the room and back. I'll stay with you."	Physically assisting the patient shows empathy.
Romberg	"Please do this, palms up. I'm right behind you if you feel unsteady. Please close your eyes and put your head back. Fine. You may open your eyes now. Please sit back down. May I help you? Let me cover you again."	Demonstrate action. Such phrases show empathy.
Kernig	"I need to uncover your leg. I'm going to bend and then straighten it. Tell me if it hurts."	
Brudzinski	"I need to put my arm under your shoulders. I'm going to move your chin down toward your chest. Just relax while I do this. Thank you."	
Diabetic testing		
Vibration	"I'm going to place this tuning fork on your toe. Please close your eyes. Do you feel anything? Please open your eyes."	
Position sense	"Now I'll move your toe. Please close your eyes. Is your toe pointing up or down? Okay, thanks. You may open your eyes."	

Table IV-3. Musculoskeletal Examination

Action	Suggested Phrasing	Comments
Wrist pain		
Inspection	"Let me take a look at your wrist and other joints."	Paraphrasing what the patient has already told you shows care and concern.
Palpation	"I know you said it hurts, so let me start with the other side. Now let me check this side."	
Range of movement	"Now I need to see how your hands are moving. Let me start with the one that doesn't hurt."	
Muscle testing for UE	"Do this. Don't let me push in. Don't let me push out. Do this. Don't let me push up. Don't let me push down. Do this. Don't let me squeeze your fingers together. Do this. Squeeze my fingers as hard as you can. Thank you."	Don't say "ouch!" if the patient squeezes too hard.
Reflexes for UE	"Now I need to tap on your arm."	Tap in three areas on each hand.
Sensory	"Now I'll check your sensation."	
Light tough	"I need to touch your hands lightly. Tell me if you feel this. Please close your eyes. Do you feel this? How about this? Does it feel the same?"	Repeat for three points on hand. Afterward, say, "Please open your eyes now."
Sharp and dull	"Now I'll check your sharp and dull touch. This is sharp. This is dull. Okay, please close your eyes. Which is this? Which is this?"	Repeat for three points on hand. Then say, "You may open your eyes now."
Tinel	"I need to tap on your wrist. Let me start with the one that doesn't hurt."	
Phalen	"Do this. Let me know if it hurts."	Demonstrate action.
Adson	"I need to take your pulse. I'm going to lift your hand. Please look at your hand. Thanks."	
Shoulder pain		
Inspection	"Let me take a look at your shoulder and other joints."	
Palpation	"I know you said it hurts, so I'll start with the other one. I need to untie your gown. Okay, now I'm going to press on your neck. Any pain? Now your shoulder blade [or] Now here. Any pain? Now let me do the same on the other side. Let me tie your gown back."	Always let the patient know beforehand when you're going to untie, raise, or lower the gown.
Range of movement	"I need to check on your shoulder movement. With the hand that doesn't hurt, do this. This. This. Now with the other hand, go only as far as you can. Do this. Do this. This. Thank you."	Repeat for other shoulder.
Muscle testing for UE	"I need to check your arm strength. Do this. Don't let me push in. Don't let me push out. Do this. Don't let me push up. Do this. Don't let me push down. Don't let me squeeze your fingers together. Do this. Squeeze my fingers as hard as you can."	
Reflexes for UE	"Now I need to tap on your arms."	Repeat for three areas.

UE = upper extremity; LE = lower extremity

(Continued)

Table IV-3. Musculoskeletal Examination (*continued*)

Action	Suggested Phrasing	Comments
Sensory for UE Light touch	"I need to check your sensation. May I pull up your sleeves? Thank you. Now I'm going to touch your hands lightly. Do you feel this? Please close your eyes. Do you feel this? And this? Does it feel the same? Do you feel this? This? Does it feel the same?"	Besides the three points on hand, check deltoid area. Repeat for four points. Then, "Please open your eyes."
Sharp and dull	"Now let's check sharp and dull. This is sharp. This is dull. Which is this? This?"	Repeat for four points. Then, "Please open your eyes."
Lower back pain Inspection	"Let me take a look at your other joints."	
Palpation	"I need to press on your back. Now I'm going to press over here. May I untie your gown?"	
Muscle testing for LE	"I need to check your leg strength. Push out. Pull back. Push on the gas [or] Push down. Pull up."	
Reflexes	"Now I'll tap on your legs."	
Sensory for LE Light touch	"I need to check your sensation. I'm going to touch your legs lightly. Do you feel this? Now please close your eyes. Do you feel this? This? Does it feel the same?"	Repeat for four points. "Open your eyes."
Sharp and dull	"Now I need to check your sharp and dull touch. This is sharp. This is dull. Okay, please close your eyes. Which is this? This?"	Repeat for four points. "Open your eyes."
Babinski	"Now I need to tickle your feet [or] I need to scratch your feet."	
Gait	"I need to see how you walk. Let me pull out the footstool. May I help you down? Please walk to the other side of the room and back. I'll be nearby."	
Range of motion	"Please bend down and try to touch your toes. Now twist from side to side [or] Do this. Now, lean back."	Demonstrate twisting.
Knee pain Inspection	"Let me check your knees."	
Palpation	"I know you said this knee hurts, so I'll start with the other one. Let me lift the sheet so I can press on your knee."	
Range of motion	"Let's see how your leg moves."	
Muscle testing for LE	"Let's check your leg strength. Push out. Pull back. Push on the gas [or] Push down. Pull up."	
Reflexes	"Now I need to tap on your legs."	
Sensory for LE Light tough	"I need to check your sensation. I'm going to touch your feet lightly. Do you feel this? Please close your eyes. Can you feel this? How about this? Is it the same? Do you feel this? This? Is it the same?"	Repeat for four points. Then, "You can open your eyes now. Thanks."
Sharp and dull	"Now let's check your sense of sharp and dull. This is sharp. This is dull. Okay, please close your eyes. Which is this? This?"	Repeat for four points. Then, "Please open your eyes."

UE = upper extremity; LE = lower extremity

(Continued)

Table IV-3. Musculoskeletal Examination (*continued*)

Action	Suggested Phrasing	Comments

Pulses
Knee joint effusion
 	
Anterior/posterior
  drawer sign
McMurray
	"I need to check your pulses."
	"Let's see if you have any swelling. Okay, now
	  the other knee."
	"I need to push and pull on your knee. Okay,
	  now the other one."
	"I'm going to push down on your knee and
	  move your foot. Okay, now the other knee."	

Collateral strain	"I need to push on your knee. Now the other one."	

Table IV-4. Cardiovascular Examination

Action	Suggested Phrasing	Comments

Sitting up
Carotid bruit
 	
Palpation of pulses
Edema
Palpation of PMI
 	
Auscultation of heart
Auscultation of lungs
	"I need to listen to your neck sounds. Please
	  take a deep breath and hold it."
	"I'm going to check your pulses."
	"I'm going to check your legs for swelling."
	"I need to lower your gown, please. I need to
	  press on your heart area."
	
	"I need to listen to your heart."
	"While you're sitting up, let me listen to
	  your lungs."
		
		For women, you may need
		  to ask, "Please lift your
		  breast. Thank you."
		Leave gown untied.
		Three levels posterior

Lying down
JVD
 	
Palpation of PMI
 	
Auscultation of heart
Costochondral
  tenderness
Epigastric
  tenderness
	"Please look to the left. I need to take a look
	  at your neck."
	"I need to press in on your heart area.
	  Let me lower your gown."
	"Let me listen to your heart."
	"Now I need to press on your chest. Any pain?"
	
	"Now I need to press on your stomach area."
		Adjust table for JVD
		  and pull out extension.
		
		Maintain eye contact.

JVD = jugular venous distention; PMI = point of maximum impulse

KAPLAN
medical

Table IV-5. Pulmonary Examination

Action	Suggested Phrasing	Comments
Posterior chest	"May I untie your gown? I need to check your lungs."	
Respiratory excursion	"Please take a deep breath. Cross your arms in front and sit up straight."	
Tactile fremitus	"Please say 99. Again."	Repeat at each level.
Percussion	"Now I'm going to tap on your chest."	
Auscultation of lungs	"I need to listen to your lungs. Please breathe in and out through your mouth. Okay, thank you."	
Anterior chest	"I need to lower your gown."	
Tactile fremitus	"Please say 99. Again."	Repeat at each level.
Percussion	"Now I'm going to tap on your chest."	
Auscultation of lungs	"Let me listen to your lungs. Please breathe in and out through your mouth. Thank you."	
Auscultation of heart	"Now I'll listen to your heart. Please breathe normally."	

Table IV-6. Abdominal Examination

Action	Suggested Phrasing	Comments
Inspection	"Let me take a look at your stomach area.	The word "abdomen" is considered medical terminology. Use "stomach area," "belly," or "tummy." If you notice any scars or abnormalities, ask about them.
Auscultation	"Now I need to listen to your belly."	Warm up your stethoscope head before touching patient with it.
Percussion	"I need to tap on your tummy."	Always examine the painful area last.
Light palpation	"I need to press lightly on your stomach area."	
Deep palpation	"I need to press a little more deeply now."	
Special tests for appendicitis Rebound tenderness Obturator sign Psoas sign CVA tenderness **Special test for cholecystitis** Murphy sign	"Now I need to press in on your stomach area. Tell me if it hurts more when I press in or let go." "I need to uncover your leg. I'm going to bend it. Tell me if it hurts." "Please turn over to your left side. I need to lift your leg and pull it back. Tell me if this is painful." "I'm going to tap on your back now. Let me know if it hurts." "I need to press in on your stomach area. Please take a deep breath and let me know if it hurts."	Because patient may be in severe pain, do this while patient is lying on left side after performing the psoas sign.

Appendix V: **Answers to Clinical Exercises and Practice Cases**

CHAPTER 3–FOCUSED MEDICAL HISTORY

Clinical Exercise 1

Compare your hypotheses for each patient presented in Clinical Exercise 1. During the CS examination, the first step of immediately generating hypotheses using the doorway information will enable you to formulate more accurate hypotheses when the patient is interviewed and examined, ultimately leading to a comprehensive differential diagnosis of each patient's problem(s).

Case A

1. Muscle contraction (tension) headache

2. Migraine headache

3. Intracerebral or subarachnoid hemorrhage

Reasoning: Although the chronology of the symptom is not yet known, common clinical problems should always be included in the initial generation of hypotheses, e.g., muscle contraction headache and migraine headache. The age of the patient with the patient's elevated blood pressure, particularly the systolic, leads to the inclusion of two types of brain hemorrhage that have an increased prevalence in patients with untreated or undertreated hypertension.

Case B

Hypotheses:

1. Upper respiratory infection

2. Acute bronchitis

3. Community-acquired pneumonia

Reasoning: It is likely this young man with a cough and an elevated temperature to 100.2 F (38 C) has either an upper or lower respiratory infection. Additional hypotheses will be generated when he presents the chronology with other dimensions of the history of the present illness.

Tip

When considering hypotheses, always list problems of varying severity.

Case C

Hypotheses:

1. Acute coronary syndrome: unstable angina or acute myocardial infarction

2. Acute infectious pleuritis, possible initial presentation of *S. pneumoniae* pneumonia

3. Musculoskeletal chest pain

Reasoning: An older man is brought to the emergency department with chest pain—the hypotheses reflect this symptom, the elevation in diastolic pressure, and the tachycardia. Remember, the cardiac rate does not provide information about the cardiac rhythm. Musculoskeletal chest pain is included because it is a common cause of anterior thoracic chest pain; however, it is placed lower on the list because all presented information suggests a more serious etiology.

Case D

Hypotheses:

1. Acute appendicitis

2. Nonspecific gastroenteritis

3. Rupture of a tubal pregnancy

Reasoning: A young woman with acute abdominal pain, a temperature of 102.1 F, and a tachycardia (likely sinus) would most likely have one of these three diagnoses because of their high incidence. Early pregnancy with a complication, e.g., rupture of a tubal pregnancy, should always be considered in the correct clinical setting.

Case E

Hypotheses:

1. Learning disability

2. Visual or auditory impairment

3. Behavioral disorder

Reasoning: During the Step 2 CS examination, concerns about an infant or child will be presented by a parent, grandparent, or guardian, either in person or via a telephone conversation. A physical examination is not conducted because the child is not present. Lack of progress in school is a common and challenging problem often presented to a physician.

Case F

Hypotheses:

1. Depression/anxiety

2. Anemia, likely iron-deficiency

3. Hypothyroidism

Reasoning: Fatigue is an extremely common concern expressed by patients. A surprising number of these patients have emotional and social reasons leading to somatic symptoms. Iron-deficiency anemia in young women is another common clinical problem, particularly in the presence of hypermenorrhea and/or several pregnancies. Hypothyroidism also has a high prevalence among patients of both sexes and all ages.

Case G

Hypotheses:

1. Acute or chronic musculoskeletal pain, i.e., lumbosacral strain

2. Intervertebral disk disease

3. Inflammatory arthropathy, e.g., ankylosing spondylitis

Reasoning: Acute or chronic lumbosacral strain is the most common cause for lower back pain. Intervertebral disk disease is certainly a common clinical problem in the right setting. Among young men, severe back pain may be the initial manifestation of the inflammatory arthropathy, ankylosing spondylitis.

Clinical Exercise 2

Remember

Mnemonic: SIQOR AAA

Case A

Site:

1. Show me where your head hurts.

Intensity/Quantity:

1. How often does the headache occur?

2. Rate this pain on a scale of 0 to 10, with 0 being no pain, and 10 being the worst pain you have experienced.

3. How do you usually tolerate pain?

Quality:

1. Describe what the pain feels like.

2. Does the pain feel like a pain you've had somewhere else?

3. When the headache moves to another spot, does it feel different?

Onset:

1. When were you last perfectly healthy?

2. When did the headache begin?

3. Have you had headaches in the past?

4. What time of day does the headache occur?

5. Where are you when the headache begins?

6. What are you doing when the pain begins?

Radiation:

1. Does the pain move to another place after it begins?

Aggravating or Alleviating factors:

1. What can increase the headache?

2. What decreases or eliminates the headache?

3. Have you tried any medication?

Associated manifestations:

1. Have you noted any other symptoms associated with the headache?

2. Do you have pain in your joints or muscles, particularly around the shoulders and joints?

3. Has your vision changed?

Case B

Site:

1. Where does the cough seem to begin—your throat or deep in your chest?

Intensity/Quantity:

1. How frequently do you cough?
2. Are you coughing up small or large amounts of fluid?
3. Is the cough getting worse or improving?

Quality:

1. Does it hurt when you cough?
2. Is the cough dry?
3. Is there any blood present in the fluid?

Onset:

1. When were you last perfectly healthy?
2. When did the cough begin?
3. Is it the first time you have had this cough?
4. What you were doing when you first noticed this cough?
5. Does the cough awaken you or in any way interfere with sleeping?
6. Do you smoke cigarettes or cigars?

Radiation:

1. Does the cough cause a problem somewhere else in your body?

Aggravating or Alleviating factors:

1. Does any position cause the cough to increase?
2. Have you done or taken anything to decrease the coughing?
3. Is the cough in any way affected by cold air?

Associated manifestations:

1. Have you had shortness of breath with the cough?
2. Your temperature is elevated today; tell me more about the fever.
3. Are you concerned about any other symptom that started with the cough?
4. Do you feel lightheaded when you cough?

Case C

Site:

1. Show me where on your chest the pain is located.

2. Do you have pain anywhere other than the chest region?

Intensity/Quantity:

1. How would you rate this pain on a scale from 1 to 10?

2. How often does the pain occur?

3. How do you usually tolerate pain?

Quality:

1. What does the pain feel like?

2. Is it there all the time?

3. Does it feel the same all the time?

Onset:

1. When did the chest pain begin?

2. Have you had the pain before?

3. If you had the pain in the past, has it changed?

4. Where were you when the pain started?

5. What were you doing when the pain started?

6. If you had the pain before, what were you doing when pain began?

Radiation:

1. Does the pain move to another place on your chest?

Aggravating or Alleviating factors:

1. Does anything you do make the pain worse?

2. Have you taken any medication to try and relieve the pain?

3. Does anything you do improve the pain?

Associated manifestations:

1. Is shortness of breath associated with the pain?

2. Have you had nausea or vomiting since the pain began?

3. Have you felt lightheaded or faint since the pain began?

Case D

Site:

1. Please point to the area that hurts. Then with one finger, if you can, point to the area that hurts the most.

2. Have you had any surgery or a medical problem in the area where the pain is located?

Intensity/Quantity:

1. On a scale of 1 to 10, how would you rate the abdominal pain?

2. Has it disappeared since starting?

3. If you've been taking your temperature, how high has it been?

Quality:

1. Can you describe the abdominal pain? For example, is it constant or does it come and go?

2. Is this a sharp pain or more like a dull throbbing pain?

3. Have you ever had pain like this before, and if you have, do you know what the problem was?

Onset:

1. When were you last perfectly fine?

2. When did the pain begin?

3. When did the fever start?

4. What were you doing when the pain started?

5. If you have been able to eat, did food increase or decrease the pain?

6. Could there be any relationship of the pain to your menstrual period?

Radiation:

1. Now point to any areas the pain moves to.

Aggravating or Alleviating factors:

1. What makes your abdomen hurt more?

2. If you took any medication for pain, did it help?

3. Does the position you are in affect your pain?

Associated manifestations:

1. Have you had any change in your bowel habits—either constipation or diarrhea?

2. Is there a possibility that you might be pregnant? (Reassure the patient that this information is sensitive, and all information will be kept confidential.)

3. Have you had shaking chills with the fever?

KAPLAN
medical

Case E

Site:

1. Has Jennifer had any complaints about any part of her body that you think might be related to the reading problem?

2. Has Jennifer's vision been tested at school or by her pediatrician?

3. Has Jennifer had many ear infections or any difficulty with her hearing?

Intensity/Quantity:

1. At what grade reading level is Jennifer?

2. How does Jennifer's reading compare with the ability of her friends?

3. How much time does Jennifer spend doing reading homework at home?

Quality:

1. Please describe what you mean by "problems learning to read"? For example, can she recognize all the words she used to, but just isn't learning new ones?

2. Does Jennifer enjoy reading?

3. Can Jennifer recognize words when someone reads to her?

Onset:

1. How long have you noticed that Jennifer has been having trouble reading?

2. When did Jennifer's teacher identify the reading problem?

3. Did Jennifer meet all the growth and development milestones when she visited the pediatrician?

4. Does Jennifer seem to read just fine at home but not in school, or vice versa?

5. Does Jennifer spontaneously pick up books, even comic books to read now? Or has she ever and doesn't any more?

6. Does Jennifer enjoy visiting the library?

Aggravating or Alleviating factors:

1. Does Jennifer seem distracted to you? For example, perhaps she is daydreaming or not paying attention?

2. Does a calm, quiet place seem to make a difference in how Jennifer is able to read or behave when she is trying to read?

3. Is Jennifer upset with herself because she is frustrated about her ability to read?

Case F

Site:

1. Does your whole body feel tired?

2. Are your muscles so weak that they cannot be moved?

3. Are you having symptoms in other part of your body?

Intensity/Quantity:

1. Does being tired prevent you from carrying out your daily activities?

2. Can you give me an idea of just how tired you are? For example, how far can you walk before you get tired, or how long can you stay awake before needing a nap?

3. Have you ever been so tired that you had to remain in bed all day?

Quality:

1. What you mean by tired?

2. Can you tell if you feel weak?

3. Does it feel like you haven't had enough sleep? Or is it more like the tiredness you feel when you have a cold or the flu?

Onset:

1. How long have you been feeling so tired?

2. Do you remember when you were last perfectly fine?

3. Is there any event or incident that you can think of that may have triggered you to feel so tired?

4. Do you feel rested and refreshed when you wake up in the morning?

5. Are you sleeping more hours than you used to?

6. What activities cause you to be the most tired?

Aggravating or Alleviating factors:

1. What makes your tiredness worse?

2. What helps to decrease your tiredness?

3. Does taking a nap during the day help?

Associated manifestations:

1. Do you have shortness of breath, either at rest or with activity?

2. Are there other symptoms you are concerned about?

3. Is there any relationship to your menstrual cycle?

Case G

Site:

1. Where in the back does it hurt?

2. Do you have any symptoms in the front of your abdomen (stomach)?

Intensity/Quantity:

1. How would you rate the severity of the pain on a scale of 1 to 10?

2. Is the pain preventing you from working?

3. Does the pain prevent you from sleeping normally?

Quality:

1. Please describe what the pain feels like to you.

2. Is the pain constant?

3. If it comes and goes, how long does it stay?

Onset:

1. When did the pain begin?

2. What were you doing when the pain started?

3. Have you ever had pain like this before?

4. When does the pain occur now?

5. Is there any relationship to the time of day?

6. Does the pain occur with a bowel movement?

Radiation:

1. Does the pain travel anywhere; for example, around to the front or down either leg?

Aggravating or Alleviating factors:

1. Which position accentuates the pain: sitting, standing, or lying down?

2. Have you tried any medication that has helped the pain?

3. Is there anything you can do to relieve the pain?

Associated manifestations:

1. Have you noticed any numbness or tingling in your legs?

2. Have you lost any feeling completely in any part of your back or legs?

3. Have you noticed any weakness in your legs?

CHAPTER 4—FOCUSED PHYSICAL EXAM

Clinical Exercise 3

Case A

Region(s) to be examined: Ms. Brown requires a rapid, efficient, and thorough neurologic examination. Practice the neurologic examination prior to the CS examination, and be prepared to carry out this examination in 7 to 8 minutes. For the mental status component, ask two questions that correlate highly with the entire mini-mental status examination: *1)* repeating and remembering three objects and *2)* serially subtracting seven starting with 100.

Case B

Region(s) to be examined: Oral cavity, pharynx, tympanic membranes, and lungs. When examining the lungs, follow the sequence of observing the symmetry of expansion, vocal fremitus, percussion, and auscultation. Both the posterior and anterior projections of the lungs are included to ensure a thorough accurate evaluation.

Case C

Region(s) to be examined: Thoracic wall, ribs, cartilages in the region of pain, lungs (same sequence as noted for patient in Case B, Mr. Muta), and heart. When examining the heart, inspect the anterior thorax for the apical impulse, palpate and identify the point of maximal impulse, and then auscultate over the four conventional valve areas. Follow and report the radiation of any murmur.

Case D

Region(s) to be examined: Carefully and gently examine the abdomen to identify areas of direct and rebound tenderness; follow the sequence of inspection, auscultation, palpation, and percussion. Auscultation is performed prior to palpation to prevent the artificial stimulation of bowel sounds if an ileus is present. The art of palpation is to use a light touch. Always percuss the superior and inferior borders of the liver—the former is best done during the examination of the anterior thorax—and report the span in centimeters measured in the right midclavicular line. Liver span by percussion in the midclavicular line is a reliable correlate of size, is related to the height of the patient, and is in the range of 8 to 12 centimeters.

Case E

Region(s) to be examined: Because the child is not present, list the physical examination as a "diagnostic test" when the note is written.

Case F

Region(s) to be examined: Facial pallor may be present. Carefully inspect the neck and palpate the thyroid gland using either the anterior, posterior, or both approaches. Remember to consider the pelvic/rectal examination as a diagnostic test.

Case G

Region(s) to be examined: The vertebral column, paraspinal musculature, and sacroiliac joints are evaluated to identify the location of the pain and determine the presence of localized tenderness. Lower limbs are examined to determine if there is nerve-root compression: pain sensation in dermatomal distributions to identify hypesthesia, and muscle power and deep tendon reflexes to aid in the location of the nerve root compression. Understand the common syndromes that affect the lower back and how to identify them on physical examination: acute and chronic lumbosacral strain, sacroiliitis, and intervertebral disc disease with nerve root compression of L5 or S1.

The musculoskeletal examination is one of the specialized examinations (the other is the neurologic examination) that should be repeatedly practiced prior to the Step 2 CS examination. Know the range of motion of joints commonly involved in clinical problems, particularly the shoulders, hip joints, knees, and ankles.

CHAPTER 5–PATIENT NOTE

Clinical Exercise 4

Practice Case 1

History

CC: Weakness and tiredness, 2–3 years

HPI: Mr. Ven, 55 years old, came in for a check-up because he feels weak and tired, even after a night of restful sleep and believes he is beginning to "feel" his age. It has come on gradually. He cannot do his usual exercise. He has also noted a weight gain of 5 pounds in the last year He is a bank vice-president and is concerned because he cannot remember the names of his clients. Mr. Venn has noticed that his right hand feels "funny," like it's asleep, especially when he first wakes up in the morning. Prior to onset of these symptoms, he had been perfectly healthy.

Physical Examination

GA: Slightly overweight man speaking in a harsh voice

VS: BP 154/96 mm Hg, pulse 48/minute; T and RR are normal

Skin: Dry and scaly front of both forearms

Neck: Thyroid gland not palpable

Heart: Apical impulse not displaced, no murmurs

Abdomen: Normal; liver span 10 cm. R midclavicular line

Right hand: Decreased pain sensation on the palm and front of thumb, index, and middle fingers

Differential Diagnosis

1. Hypothyroidism (with carpal tunnel syndrome)
2. Iron-deficiency versus macrocytic anemia
3. Anxiety with depression
4. Metastatic carcinoma
5. Structural brain disease

Diagnostic Workup

1. CBC, electrolytes
2. Rectal examination and analysis
3. Serum TSH
4. Fecal occult blood
5. CT scan of head

Practice Case 2

History

CC:	42-year-old female c/o chest pain

HPI: Began 10 hours ago. Constant, sharp pain across chest. Pain 5/10. No radiation. No shortness of breath or palpitations. Not relieved or aggravated by food, exercise, or deep inspiration.

PMH: No previous h/o chest pain; no HTN, heart disease

FH: No h/o heart disease or similar chest pain

OB/GYN: LMP 2 weeks ago, regular

SEX HX: Sexually active with husband only. No h/o STDs

SH: Nonsmoker; drinks ETOH 2 glasses wine/week

Physical Examination

VS: WNL except BP 150/90 mm Hg

CV: S1/S2 normal, no murmurs, rubs or gallop; no JVD

Chest: Clear to auscultation BL, tactile fremitus normal, no dullness to percussion, no clubbing, no cyanosis; pain on sternal palpation

ABD: Bowl sounds present; no pain on palpation

Differential Diagnosis

1. MI (acute: pain constant but radiates with diaphoresis)
2. Angina (unstable)
3. Costochondritis (tenderness on palpation of costochondral junction, pleuritic)
4. Pneumothorax (pleuritic, radiates)
5. GERD

Diagnostic Workup

1. CPK-MB, troponin
2. EKG
3. CXR, abdominal x-ray
4. Echocardiogram
5. EGD

Practice Case 3

History

CC: 58-year-old male c/o L knee and L great toe pain

HPI: Woke 5 hours ago by burning L knee and L great toe pain, rapidly intensified to 9/10. No radiation. Associated with hotness to touch and swelling of areas. Aggravated by weight of bedclothes on leg. Ibuprofen alleviated pain to 5/10 and swelling. No h/o fever, trauma, arthritis or migratory joint pains.

PMH: H/o milder, shorter R great toe pain 4 hours ago after son's wedding. Ibuprofen alleviated pain. No h/o HTN, DM, renal or ischemic heart disease. Mildly obese. NKA. Meds: occasional ibuprofen and acetaminophen.

FH: No h/o arthritis or joint problems; father died 10 years ago of lung cancer

SEX Hx: Sexually active with wife only. No h/o STDs.

SH: Office supervisor, mostly seated at work. Stopped smoking 10 years ago. Irregularly drinks ETOH. 1 day ago drank 5 beers and ate plenty of meats.

Physical Examination

VS: WNL except T: 99.8 F; RR: 16/min

Musculoskeletal: (−) Lesions or scars on L lower ext.

      (+) L knee and L great toe tenderness

      Painful limited flexions/extension of L knee and L great toe

      Warm on L or R lower ext.

      Swelling of L or R lower ext.

      Sharp/dull intact muscle strength and reflexes equal WNL BL

      Pedal pulses equal WNL BL

Differential Diagnosis

1. Acute gout
2. Pseudogout
3. Septic arthritis
4. Rheumatoid arthritis
5. Osteoarthritis

Diagnostic Workup

1. X-ray of L knee and L great toe
2. L knee/L great toe arthrocentesis
3. Joint fluid analysis (cell count, Gram stain, polarized light microscopy)
4. CBC, differential, ESR, BUN, creatinine, serum uric acid, rheumatoid factor

Practice Case 4

History

CC: 58 yo M c/o severe chest pain

HPI: Began 1 h ago following strenuous activity, as sharp substernal chest pain 7/10, that does not radiate. Associated SOB, no sweating, nausea. Not relieved by rest.

PMH: No previous h/o chest pain. Meds: vitamins, NKA, healthy diet with no weight changes

FH: Father deceased age 67 of "heart trouble"

Sex Hx: Sexually active with wife only. No h/o STDs

SH: Retired, nonsmoker, no h/o ETOH

Physical Examination

VS: WNL, except HR: 110/min, RR: 22/min

Chest: Clear to auscultation B/L, no pain on palpation, tactile fremitus normal

CV: S1/S2 normal, no murmurs, rubs, or gallops; no JVD, no peripheral edema, clubbing or cyanosis

ABD: Bowel sounds present, tympanic in all 4 quadrants, no palpable masses or pain on palpation

Differential Diagnosis

1. MI
2. Angina
3. Hypertrophic cardiomyopathy
4. Pericarditis
5. Esophageal spasm

Diagnostic Workup

1. CPK-MB, troponin, ABG, CBC
2. EKG
3. CXR
4. Echocardiogram
5. Esophageal manometry

Practice Case 5

History

CC: 48 yo F c/o confusion, blurry vision, and SOB

HPI: Insidious onset of dyspnea, blurry vision, and difficulty thinking starting 3 h ago while at sedentary office job. No known precipitating or alleviating factors. Associated headache, dizziness, and mild palpitations. No fever, nausea, or vomiting

PMH: HTN, no other known cardiovascular, lung or vision disorders. Meds: thiazide diuretic, NKA, healthy diet with no weight changes or sleep problems

FH: No h/o heart or lung problems or HTN

OB/GYN: LMP 2 weeks ago, regular, g2, p2

Sex Hx: Not sexually active. No h/o STDs

SH: Nonsmoker, occasional ETOH 1 glass of wine/month

Physical Examination

VS: WNL, except RR: 16/min, BP: 230/150 mm Hg

HEENT: PERLA, EOMs WNL, no visual field defects or eyeball prominence, sharp disc margins, normal vasculature

CV: S1/S2 normal, no murmurs, rubs, or gallop, no JVD, no peripheral edema

Neuro: CN II–XII intact, DTR 2+ symmetric, sharp/dull intact, muscle strength equal and WNL B/L

Differential Diagnosis

1. Hypertensive crisis
2. Angina
3. Cerebrovascular accident
4. Intraparenchymal brain hemorrhage
5. Aortic dissection

Diagnostic Workup

1. CPK-MB, troponin, BUN, creatinine
2. EKG
3. CT scan head
4. Echocardiogram

CHAPTER 6—CLINICAL PRACTICE CASES

Practice Case 1

Standardized Patient History-Taking Checklist

1. Where is the **S**ite of the pain?

2. What is the **I**ntensity of the pain and cough? Are they getting worse?

3. How would you describe the pain and cough (**Q**uality)? Is the cough productive?

4. When did the cough and associated symptoms begin (**O**nset)?

5. Does the chest pain **R**adiate? Is it associated with coughing?

6. Is the cough **A**ssociated with fever, chills, night sweats, weight loss, or hemoptysis?

7. Does anything **A**lleviate or **A**ggravate the symptoms?

8. Have you had this before or known anyone with similar symptoms?

9. Do you have a history of lung disease?

10. Do you take any medications?

11. Any HIV risk factors (sex with men or without condoms, sex with commercial sex workers, intravenous drug use, other exposures)?

12. Do you smoke, drink, or use illicit drugs?

13. Does anyone in your family have any major illness or similar symptoms?

14. Have you traveled anywhere outside the country?

Standardized Patient Physical Examination Checklist

1. Examinee washes hands *prior* to examination.

2. Examinee evaluates oropharynx for thrush and/or other lesions.

3. Examinee auscultates lungs.

4. Examinee palpates lungs for tactile fremitus.

5. Examinee percusses lungs.

6. Examinee performs lymph node exam.

7. Examinee auscultates precordium in at least two positions.

8. Examinee percusses abdomen in all four quadrants.

9. Examinee auscultates abdomen.

10. Examinee palpates abdomen in all four quadrants.

11. Examinee examines skin for any rash and/or other lesions.

12. Examinee examines extremities for edema/clubbing/cyanosis.

History

CC: 52 y/o M c/o cough, fatigue, and chest pain

HPI   • Started with cough insidiously ~6 months ago

     • Progressive, getting worse, now with CP

     • Associated with rare hemoptysis, fatigue, night sweats ×1 month

     • 20-lb wt loss over 4 months + anorexia

     • Chest pain ×2–3 days, right-sided, 4/10 intensity, sharp and pleuritic, nonradiating, partial relief with acetaminophen

     • No orthopnea/SOB/nausea/diaphoresis

Remember

Kaplan Medical Mnemonic

SIQOR AAA

PMH:
- Unclear h/o recurrent lung infections
- Meds: acetaminophen, OTC cough suppressant, NKDA

FH:
- Parents alive and well, no known familial illnesses

Sex Hx:
- (+) sex w/men
- (+) h/o of STDs

SH:
- (+) cig, 35–70 pack-year
- (+) IVDU, heroin
- ETOH
- Recent incarceration/sick contact in prison

Physical Examination

VS: Febrile at 100.8 F, mild tachypnea with RR: 22/min, Po_2: 92% on RA, otherwise WNL

HEENT: Oropharynx/oral cavity clear, no erythema, ulcers or thrush. No cervical/supraclavicular or axillary lymphadenopathy

Chest: Clear to auscultation and percussion B/L, no pain on palpation, tactile fremitus WNL, (+) cough on expiration, (+) pleuritic pain

CV: S1/S2 normal, no M/R/G, no JVD, no peripheral edema, clubbing, or cyanosis

Abd: Soft, nontender, nondistended, normal BS, tympanic in all 4 quadrants, no masses or HSM present

Skin: Tattoo on left shoulder, two reddish-purple macules left shin

Differential Diagnosis

1. Pulmonary TB (prison, HIV risk factors, hemoptysis, night sweats, weight loss, fatigue, pleurisy)
2. *Pneumocystis carinii* pneumonia (HIV risk factors = sex with men, IVDU, prison tattoo, insidious onset of dry, hacking cough, pleurisy)
3. Pneumonia (community acquired versus atypical organisms)
4. Lung cancer
5. Chronic bronchitis

Diagnostic Workup

1. CXR, CT scan (if CXR nonrevealing)
2. Place PPD with controls
3. HIV test (Western blot and ELISA)
4. Sputum induction for culture, Gram stain, PCP analysis (silver or Giemsa stain), and acid-fast bacillus smear ×3
5. Blood cultures ×2, WBC with differential

Practice Case 2

Standardized Patient History-Taking Checklist

1. Where is the **Site** of the pain?
2. What is the **Intensity** of the pain?
3. How would you describe the pain (**Quality**)?
4. When did the pain begin (**Onset**)?
5. Does the stomach pain **Radiate**?
6. Is the pain related to eating?
7. Is the pain **Associated** with nausea/vomiting/hematemesis/melena/hematochezia?
8. Does anything **Alleviate** the symptoms?
9. Does anything **Aggravate** the symptoms?
10. Have you had this before?
11. Do you take any medications, specifically NSAIDs or antacids?
12. Do you smoke, drink, or use illicit drugs?
13. Does anyone in your family have any major illness or similar symptoms?
14. Do you have any cardiac risk factors (family history of cardiac disease, hyperlipidemia, diabetes)?
15. What is your diet like?

Standardized Patient Physical Examination Checklist

1. Examinee washes hands *prior* to examination.
2. Examinee auscultates lungs.
3. Examinee palpates lungs for tactile fremitus.
4. Examinee auscultates precordium in at least two positions.
5. Examinee examines neck for presence of JVD.
6. Examinee auscultates abdomen.
7. Examinee percusses abdomen in all four quadrants.
8. Examinee palpates abdomen in all four quadrants.
9. Examinee examines extremities for edema/clubbing/cyanosis.

History

CC: 31 yo M c/o chest/abdominal pain

HPI: • 1 y h/o epigastric pain (**Site**)
        • Pain rated 4/10 (**Intensity/Quantity**)
        • Burning **Quality**, insidious **Onset**
        • **Radiates** from epigastrium to back
        • **Associated** with reflux symptoms, dark stools
        • **Alleviated** with food and antacids, unrelated to exertion
        • **Aggravated** by alcohol
        • Denies SOB, nausea, vomiting, weight loss, fever, chills, night sweats, weight change, hematochezia

PMH:
- No previous episodes of current symptoms
- NKDA
- Uses OTC antacids, denies any other medications or NSAID use
- No h/o diabetes, cardiac disease, hyperlipidemia
- Erratic, high-fat diet

FH:
- No family h/o cardiac or gastric disease

SH:
- Type A personality
- (+) ETOH 1–2 drinks (gin)/day
- (+) 20 pack-year tobacco use
- No drug use

Physical Examination

VS: Tachycardic at 108/min; otherwise within normal limits

Gen: No acute distress, pale

Chest: Clear to auscultation B/L, tactile fremitus normal

CV: S1/S2 normal, no murmurs/rubs/gallops, no JVD, no peripheral edema, cyanosis, clubbing

Abd: Mild tenderness to palpation epigastrium, no guarding or rebound tenderness. Bowel sounds present, tympanic in all four quadrants; no palpable masses or pain on palpation; negative Murphy sign

Differential Diagnosis

1. Peptic ulcer disease (PUD)
2. GERD (without PUD)
3. Chronic pancreatitis
4. Alcohol-induced gastritis
5. Anginal equivalent

Diagnostic Workup

1. Rectal exam
2. Stool exam for occult blood
3. WBC, hematocrit, amylase, lipase, BUN, creatinine, CK, CK-MB, troponin, type and cross blood
4. Upper endoscopy
5. EKG

Practice Case 3

Standardized Patient History-Taking Checklist

1. Where is the **S**ite of the pain?
2. What is the **I**ntensity of the pain?
3. How would you describe the pain (**Q**uality)?
4. When did the pain begin (**O**nset)?
5. Does the pain **R**adiate?
6. Is the pain **A**ssociated with urination?
7. Does anything **A**lleviate the symptoms?
8. Does anything **A**ggravate the symptoms?
9. Have you had this before?
10. What does your blood pressure normally run?
11. Have you had urinary infections or kidney stones in the past?
12. Do you suffer from diabetes?
13. Do you smoke, drink, or use illicit drugs?
14. Does anyone in your family have any major illness?
15. Have you suffered from dehydration (reduced fluids, increased sweating, etc.)?
16. Is your diabetes under good control?

Standardized Patient Physical Examination Checklist

1. Examinee washes hands *prior* to examination.
2. Examinee auscultates lungs.
3. Examinee auscultates precordium in at least two positions.
4. Examinee examines neck for evaluation of jugular venous pressure.
5. Examinee auscultates abdomen.
6. Examinee percusses abdomen in all four quadrants.
7. Examinee palpates abdomen in all four quadrants.
8. Examinee checks for costovertebral angle tenderness.
9. Examinee examines extremities for edema/clubbing/cyanosis.
10. Examinee comments on the patient's near fall; encourages patient to lie down.

History

CC: 63 yo F back pain, fever

HPI:
- 3 days ago, fatigue, nausea, urinary frequency
- 2 days ago, developed fevers, chills, back pain, myalgias/arthralgia, headaches
- Pain localized to back, suprapubic area, 4/10 intensity
- Pain is dull, constant
- Mild relief with acetaminophen; otherwise, no clear precipitating, alleviating, or exacerbating factors.
- No vomiting (tolerating po diet), weight loss, hematuria
- Recent reduced fluid intake

PMH: • Previous history of somewhat similar UTI symptoms (current episode worse)

• Allergies: NKDA

• Current meds:

    – Acetaminophen

    – Metformin (off ×3 days)

    – Lisinopril (off ×3 days)

• History of NIDDM, recurrent UTIs, renal calculi, hypertension, foot ulcer

FH: • Mother with DM

SH: • No ETOH, drugs, tobacco

Physical Examination

VS: Remarkable for fever of 101.1 F, relative hypotension (normally hypertensive) of 115/80 mm Hg, and tachycardia of 108/min

Gen: Anxious, mild distress, warm and flushed

Chest: Clear to auscultation B/L, tactile fremitus normal

CV: S1/S2 normal, no murmurs/rubs/gallops, no JVD, no peripheral edema, cyanosis or clubbing

Abd: Mild suprapubic tenderness, no guarding or rebound tenderness. Bowel sounds present, tympanic in all four quadrants, no palpable masses or pain on palpation. (–) Murphy sign, (+) R CVA tenderness

Differential Diagnosis

1. Pyelonephritis
2. Urosepsis
3. Nephrolithiasis
4. Diabetic cytopathy
5. Ovarian torsion or cyst

Diagnostic Workup

1. GU/pelvic and rectal examination
2. Microscopic urinalysis and urine culture
3. WBC, hematocrit, blood cultures ×2, BUN, creatinine
4. KUB
5. If above not revealing, then IVP or noncontrast CT scan

Practice Case 4

Standardized Patient History-Taking Checklist

1. When did this start?
2. How much and how often have you bled?
3. Is there any pain or discomfort?
4. Have you had any lightheadedness, dizziness, unstable gait, loss of consciousness, palpitations, or difficulty thinking clearly (evidence of severe blood loss)?
5. Have you ever had a colonoscopy or flexible sigmoidoscopy (colon cancer screening)?
6. Any history of dark stools?
7. Have you had any fevers, chills, or sick contacts?
8. What does your blood pressure normally run?
9. Have you ever bled before (**Previous episode**)?
10. Are you allergic to any medications (**Allergies**)?
11. Do you take any medications, NSAIDs specifically (**Medicines**)?
12. What other medical illnesses and hospitalizations have you had (**History**)?
13. Have you had urinary or gastrointestinal changes (**Review of systems**)?
14. Does anyone in your family have cancer or any major illnesses (**Family history**)?
15. Do you smoke, drink, or use illicit drugs (**Social history**)?

Standardized Patient Physical Examination Checklist

1. Examinee washes hands *prior* to examination.
2. Examinee auscultates lungs.
3. Examinee auscultates precordium in at least two positions.
4. Examinee examines neck for evaluation of jugular venous pressure.
5. Examinee auscultates abdomen.
6. Examinee percusses abdomen in all four quadrants.
7. Examinee palpates abdomen in all four quadrants.
8. Examinee asks if abdominal scar is related to previous operation.
9. Examinee examines extremities for edema/clubbing/cyanosis.

History

CC: 72 yo F c/o hematochezia

HPI:
- Bright red blood per rectum ×1 day
- 4 bowel movements, each filling toilet with blood
- No pain/cramping
- Associated with feeling of weakness, dizziness
- (–) Fever, chills, nausea, vomiting, melena, weight loss, change in bowel movements

PMH:
- Allergies: NKDA
- Medications: HCTZ, MVI, acetaminophen PRN; denies NSAID use
- No previous bleeding, h/o HTN, osteoporosis, diverticulitis, cholecystectomy
- No dietary changes, sick contacts
- No prior colonoscopy or colon cancer screening

Remember

Kaplan Mnemonic
PAM HR FOSS

FH: Noncontributory, no FH of bleeding/GI malignancy

SH: No ETOH/cig/drug use

Physical Examination

VS: Afebrile, relative hypotension (h/o HTN) at 108/55 mm Hg, tachycardic at 108/min

Gen: Well appearing, no apparent distress

Chest: Clear to auscultation B/L

CV: Tachycardic and regular rhythm, no murmurs/rubs/gallops, JVP <5 cm

Abd: Surgical scar consistent with cholecystectomy, no other skin lesions; + bowel sounds, abd tympanic to percussion all 4 quadrants, no hepatosplenomegaly. No palpable masses, soft, nontender, nondistended. No guarding or rebound tenderness.

Differential Diagnosis

1. Diverticulosis
2. Brisk upper GI bleed (i.e., PUD)
3. Internal hemorrhoids, arterial-venous malformation (or other lower GI bleed source)
4. Infectious diarrhea (*E. coli*, *Campylobacter*)
5. Colon cancer or other malignancy (usually slow bleed)

Diagnostic Workup

1. Rectal exam
2. Hematocrit, serum sodium, potassium, chloride, bicarbonate, BUN, creatinine, type and cross blood
3. Nasogastric lavage (rule out upper GI source)
4. Colonoscopy (upper endoscopy if lavage positive); barium study if not available
5. Stool cultures

Practice Case 5

Standardized Patient History-Taking Checklist

1. Where is the pain located (**Site**)?
2. What is the **Intensity** of the pain on a scale from 1 to 10?
3. How would you describe the pain (**Quality**)?
4. Are you aware of anything that might have brought this on (**Onset**)?
5. Does the pain move (**Radiate**)?
6. SOB? Sweating? Nausea or vomiting (**Associated manifestations**)?
7. Does anything make the pain better (**Alleviating factors**)?
8. Does anything make the pain worse (**Aggravating factors**)?
9. Specifically, is the pain worse with inspiration or movement?
10. Have you ever had this or a similar experience before?
11. Do you have a history of diabetes, high cholesterol, blood clots, or bleeding disorders?
12. Have you recently been immobilized (international flight, recent operation, etc.)?
13. Do you take any medications?
14. Specifically, do you take oral contraceptive pills?
15. Are you currently sexually active?
16. Is there a history of smoking, drinking, or drug use?
17. Does anyone in your family have similar problems or related illness/conditions?

Standardized Patient Physical Examination Checklist

1. Examinee washes hands *prior* to examination.
2. Examinee auscultates lungs in all lung fields.
3. Examinee percusses lung fields.
4. Examinee palpates lungs for tactile fremitus.
5. Examinee looks for pain with inspiration and positional changes.
6. Examinee evaluates neck for JVD.
7. Examinee auscultates precordium in at least two positions.
8. Examinee percusses abdomen in all four quadrants.
9. Examinee auscultates abdomen.
10. Examinee palpates abdomen in all four quadrants.
11. Examinee examines extremities for edema/clubbing/cyanosis and varicose veins/cords for lower extremities.

History

CC: 48 yo F c/o chest pain

HPI: • Chest pain ×4 hours
         • 6/10, sharp
         • Sudden onset
         • No radiation
         • No relief with acetaminophen, worse with deep breaths
         • Denies nausea/vomiting/diaphoresis/fevers/chills/cough

PMH:
- No previous episodes of chest pain
- Allergies: NKDA
- Medications: oral contraceptive pill, acetaminophen PRN, MVI
- H/o HTN, appendectomy
- No urinary complaints, GI changes, leg pain or swelling

FH: No early heart disease or other illnesses

SH:
- No ETOH/drug use
- (+) Tobacco use, approx. 15-pack-year history
- Sexually active with husband, monogamous

Physical Examination

VS: Low-grade fever at 100.4 F, tachycardic 109/min, tachypneic at 26/min

Gen: Anxious, mild distress

Chest: Pain with inspiration, nonlabored breathing; RR of 25 to 30/min. Clear to auscultation and percussion B/L. No cyanosis/clubbing. Nontender to palpation. No rales, wheezes, rubs, or rhonchi. No dullness to percussion. Tactile fremitus within normal limits.

CV: Normal S1, S2. Pulses 2+ B/L. Point of maximum impulse nondisplaced; tachycardic rate and regular rhythm, no murmurs/rubs/gallops, JVP <5 cm

Abd: Surgical scar consistent with appendectomy; no other skin lesions. + BS, abd tympanic to percussion all 4 quadrants, no hepatosplenomegaly. No palpable masses, soft, nontender, nondistended.

Differential Diagnosis

1. Pulmonary embolus
2. Myocardial infarction
3. Spontaneous pneumothorax
4. Pneumonia
5. Muscle strain

Diagnostic Workup

1. CXR (PA and lateral)
2. WBC with differential, D-dimer
3. $\dot{V}/\dot{Q}$ scan (or CT angiography)
4. EKG, consider stress test if abnormal
5. CK, CK-MB, troponin

Practice Case 6

Standardized Patient History-Taking Checklist

1. Where is the headache located? (**Site**)
2. How severe is the headache? Is it the worst of your life? (**Intensity/Quantity**)
3. Can you describe the headache? (**Quality**)
4. What were you doing when the headache started? (**Onset**)
5. Does the pain move anywhere? (**Radiation**)
6. Are you nauseous? Did you lose consciousness, suffer from seizure, or have any visual disturbances/pain with looking at lights? (**Associated manifestations**)
7. Did anything make the pain better? (**Alleviating factors**)
8. Did anything make the pain worse? (**Aggravating factors**)
9. Do you suffer from headaches regularly or recently? (**Previous episode**)
10. Are you allergic to any medications? (**Allergies**)
11. Do you take any medications, specifically cold remedies and diet pills? (**Medicines**)
12. What other medical illnesses and hospitalizations have you had? Have you had any fevers, chills, sick contacts, or recent colds? (**History**)
13. Does anyone in your family have any major illnesses? (**Family history**)
14. Do you smoke, drink, or use illicit drugs? When? (**Social history**)
15. Are you sexually active? (**Sexual history**)

Standardized Patient Physical Examination Checklist

1. Examinee washes hands *prior* to examination.
2. Examinee determines patient's mental status and level of alertness.
3. Examinee performs funduscopic examination.
4. Examinee performs cranial nerve examination.
5. Examinee checks motor strength.
6. Examinee checks deep tendon reflexes.
7. Examinee evaluates sensation with at least two modalities (sharp, dull, proprioceptive).
8. Examinee checks cerebellar function (dysmetria, dysdiadochokinesia, or Romberg).
9. Examinee performs Babinski test.
10. Examinee performs either Kernig or Brudzinski test.
11. Examinee auscultates lungs.
12. Examinee auscultates precordium in at least two positions.
13. Examinee auscultates abdomen.
14. Examinee palpates abdomen in all four quadrants.
15. Examinee examines extremities for edema/clubbing/cyanosis.

History

CC: 29 yo M c/o headache

HPI: • Onset while at rest, woke from sleep
      • Sharp, rated 10/10; "worst headache of life"
      • Radiates down neck and spine

- • (+) Nausea
- • (–) Loss of consciousness, fevers, chills, seizures, confusion, URI sx
- • No relief with OTC pain meds
- • Worse with cough/head movement

PMH:
- • One headache 1 day prior to admission
- • Allergies: NKDA
- • Medications: no regular meds; denies cold remedies, diet pills
- • No previous illness or hospitalizations

FH:
- • Uncle on dialysis for polycystic kidney disease
- • No h/o CVA, CAD, vascular disease

Sex Hx: Sexually active with wife, no other partners, no h/o STD

SH:
- • (+) Alcohol, daily use
- • (+) Cig, 10-pack/year history
- • (+) Nasal cocaine, (–) IVDU

Physical Examination

VS: Low-grade fever at 100 F, hypertensive and bradycardic, 169/108 mm Hg and 48/min

Gen: Moderate distress, uncomfortable

Ophth: EOMI, PERRL, (+) photophobia, no papilledema or funduscopic abnormalities

Neuro: A&O ×2 (cannot recall date); CN II–XII intact; motor 5/5 all muscle groups; DTRs 2+ symmetric; sensation intact to sharp, dull, and proprioceptive stimuli. (–) Romberg, no dysmetria, (–) Babinski, (+) Kernig, (+) Brudzinski

Chest: Clear to auscultation B/L

CV: Bradycardic rate and regular rhythm, no murmurs/rubs/gallops, JVP <5 cm

Abd: Soft, nontender, nondistended, no palpable masses +BS

Differential Diagnosis

1. Ruptured berry aneurysm
2. Cocaine-induced hypertensive intracerebral hemorrhage
3. Meningitis (bacterial vs. viral)
4. Embolic hemorrhagic infarction (i.e., endocarditis)
5. Carotid dissection

Diagnostic Workup

1. CT scan
2. Lumbar puncture (if negative)
3. CSF cultures/Gram stain, cell count, protein, and glucose
4. WBC with differential, PT (with INR), PTT, blood cultures
5. MRI/MRA (if previous imaging studies negative)

Practice Case 7

Standardized Patient History-Taking Checklist

1. Where is the pain located? (**S**ite)
2. On a scale of 1 to 10, how severe is the pain? (**I**ntensity/Quantity)
3. Can you describe the pain? Is it sharp, dull, throbbing, etc.? (**Q**uality)
4. What were you doing when the pain started? (**O**nset)
5. Does the pain move anywhere? (**R**adiation)
6. Are you nauseous? Did you vomit, notice any change in your stools, or difficulty breathing? (**A**ssociated manifestations)
7. Did anything make the pain better? (**A**lleviating factors)
8. Did anything make the pain worse? (**A**ggravating factors)
9. Has anything like this happened before? (**P**revious episode)
10. Are you allergic to any medications? (**A**llergies)
11. Do you take any medications? (**M**edicines)
12. What other medical illnesses and hospitalizations have you had? Have you had any fevers, chills, sick contacts, weight loss, or dietary changes? (**H**istory)
13. Does anyone in your family have any major illnesses? (**F**amily history)
14. When was your last menstrual period? (**O**b/Gyn)
15. Do you smoke, drink, or use illicit drugs? (**S**ocial history)
16. When was your last drink?
17. Are you sexually active? Condoms? (**S**exual history)

Standardized Patient Physical Examination Checklist

1. Examinee washes hands *prior* to examination.
2. Examinee auscultates lungs.
3. Examinee auscultates precordium in at least two positions
4. Examinee examines neck for evaluation of jugular venous pressure.
5. Examinee inspects abdomen for skin discoloration.
6. Examinee auscultates abdomen.
7. Examinee percusses abdomen in all four quadrants.
8. Examinee palpates abdomen in all four quadrants.
9. Examinee checks for Murphy sign.
10. Examinee checks for Rovsing, obturator, or iliopsoas signs.
11. Examinee examines extremities for edema/clubbing/cyanosis.

History

CC: 31 y/o F c/o abdominal pain

HPI: • 5 hours abdominal pain
       • Epigastric/RUQ → back
       • Aching, "band-like", 10/10
       • (+) Nausea/emesis ×3 (no blood), (+) SOB
       • (−) Recent fevers, chills, cough, dysuria, diarrhea, melena, sick contacts

- Improved with position (leaning forward)
- Worse when recumbent position

PMH:
- Previous episode abd pain requiring ICU stay
- Allergies: NKDA
- Medications: none
- Past h/o alcoholism, gallstones, UTIs

FH:
- Mother with DM
- Father with HTN
- Parents alive and well

Sex Hx: No STDs, monogamous, condoms

Ob/Gyn: No children, LMP 2 weeks ago

SH:
- (+) ETOH, last drink approx. 4 hours ago, 1/5 vodka, drinks daily
- (−) cig/tob
- Unemployed

Physical Examination

VS: Febrile at 101.0 F, borderline BP at 102/60 mm Hg, tachycardic at 109/min, tachypneic at 27/min

Gen: Anxious, uncomfortable, moderate distress

Chest: Clear to auscultation B/L

CV: Tachycardic rate and regular rhythm, no murmurs/rubs/gallops, JVP <5 cm. No peripheral edema.

Abd: No skin lesions or surgical scars; + bowel sounds, abd tympanic to percussion all 4 quadrants, no hepatosplenomegaly or palpable masses; (+) guarding, (−) rebound, tender to palpation in epigastrium and RUQ; (−) Murphy, (−) Rovsing, (−) iliopsoas, (−) obturator sign

Differential Diagnosis

1. Pancreatitis, alcoholic vs. biliary
2. Alcohol-induced gastritis vs. peptic ulcer disease
3. Cholecystitis
4. Appendicitis
5. PID, ectopic pregnancy

Diagnostic Workup

1. Rectal (with stool occult blood exam) and pelvic exam
2. Amylase, lipase, WBC with differential, BUN, creatinine, calcium, LDH, glucose, beta-HCG
3. CT scan of abdomen/pelvis with contrast
4. Ultrasound (if poor visualization of appendix and biliary structures with CT)
5. Endoscopy (if previous studies unrevealing)

KAPLAN
medical

Practice Case 8

Standardized Patient History-Taking Checklist

1. Where is the pain located (**S**ite)?
2. What is the **I**ntensity (quantity) of the pain?
3. How would you describe the pain (**Q**uality)?
4. When did the pain begin (**O**nset)?
5. Does the pain **R**adiate?
6. Is the pain **A**ssociated with urination? Fevers? Back pain?
7. Does anything **A**lleviate the symptoms?
8. Does anything **A**ggravate the symptoms?
9. Have you had this before? (**P**revious episode)
10. Do you have any drug **A**llergies?
11. Do you take any **M**edications?
12. Have you had any previous **H**istory of hospitalizations or medical illnesses?
13. Do you have pain with urination, blood in your urine, the need to urinate immediately, or urinary frequency (**R**eview of systems)?
14. Have you had diarrhea, nausea, or vomiting (Review of systems)?
15. Does anyone in your family have any major illness (**F**amily history)?
16. When was your last menstrual period (**O**b/Gyn history)?
17. Do you smoke, drink, or use illicit drugs (**S**ocial history)?
18. Do you have sex? Use condoms? History of STDs (**S**exual history)?

Standardized Patient Physical Examination Checklist

1. Examinee washes hands *prior* to examination.
2. Examinee auscultates lungs.
3. Examinee auscultates precordium in at least two positions.
4. Examinee auscultates abdomen.
5. Examinee percusses abdomen in all four quadrants.
6. Examinee palpates abdomen in all four quadrants.
7. Examinee specifically palpates and percusses the bladder (lower abd/pelvis).
8. Examinee palpates for costovertebral angle tenderness.
9. Examinee examines extremities for edema/clubbing/cyanosis.

History

CC: 19 yo F abd pain

HPI:
- Lower abdominal pain ×1 day
- 4/10 with no radiation
- (+) Dysuria, (+) urgency, (+) frequency, (+) cloudy urine
- (−) Fever, chills, back pain, GI sx, vaginal discharge
- Pain worse with urination, little relief with acetaminophen/cranberry juice

PMH:
- No prior occurrences
- Allergies: NKDA
- Medications: none
- No prior medical history/hospitalizations

Remember

- SIQOR AAA
- PAM HR FOSS

KAPLAN
medical

FH: Mom: HTN, no known familial illnesses

Sex H: • Sex with boyfriend, no condoms

          • No h/o STD

          • Recently became sexually active

SH: • Rare ETOH (social use at parties)

             No cig/drug use

Physical Examination

VS: Within normal limits

Gen: Well appearing, NAD

Chest: Clear to auscultation, B/L

CV: Regular rate and rhythm, no murmurs/rubs/gallops

Abd: (+) BS, abd tympanic to percussion all 4 quadrants, no hepatosplenomegaly. No pal-
           pable masses; soft, nondistended. Mild tenderness to palpation lower mid abdomen.
           No guarding or rebound tenderness.

Differential Diagnosis

1. Acute cystitis ("honeymoon cystitis," likely *Staphylococcus saprophyticus*)
2. Pyelonephritis
3. Cervicitis (chlamydial vs. *Neisseria gonorrhoeae*)/vaginitis
4. Gastroenteritis
5. Ectopic vs. intrauterine pregnancy

Diagnostic Workup

1. Dipstick urinalysis +/– urine culture (culture not required for most cystitis)
2. Pelvic exam
3. Pap smear, cervical swab for gonorrhea and chlamydia
4. Urine beta-hCG
5. WBC, BUN, creatinine

Practice Case 9

Standardized Patient History-Taking Checklist

1. When did this start?
2. How often do you go to the bathroom?
3. Is there any pain or discomfort?
4. Do you have difficulty initiating or stopping urination? Forcefully urinating?
5. Have you ever noticed blood in your urine?
6. Any weight loss, anorexia, body or back pain?
7. Have you suffered fevers, chills, or a penile discharge?
8. Have you ever bled before?
9. Are you allergic to any medications?
10. Do you take any medications?
11. What other medical illnesses and hospitalizations have you had?
12. Does anyone in your family have cancer or any major illnesses?
13. Do you smoke, drink, or use illicit drugs?
14. Are you sexually active?
15. Have you ever had any sexually transmitted diseases?

Standardized Patient Physical Examination Checklist

1. Examinee washes hands *prior* to examination.
2. Examinee auscultates lungs.
3. Examinee auscultates precordium in at least two positions.
4. Examinee auscultates abdomen.
5. Examinee percusses abdomen in all four quadrants.
6. Examinee palpates abdomen in all four quadrants.
7. Examinee specifically palpates and percusses the bladder (lower abd/pelvis).
8. Examinee checks for costovertebral angle tenderness.
9. Examinee examines extremities for edema/clubbing/cyanosis.
10. Examinee tests lower extremity strength.
11. Examinee tests lower extremity sensation.
12. Examinee tests DTRs and/or Babinski sign.

History

CC: 65 yo M c/o difficulty sleeping

HPI: • 2-year h/o nocturia, 3–4× per night
  • (+) Frequency, (+) hesitancy, (+) weak stream
  • (−) Gross hematuria, dysuria, fevers, chills, weight loss, body/back pain, nausea
  • No relief with PM po fluid restriction
  • No exacerbating factors
  • Progressive, insidious onset

PMH: • No previous urinary problems

• Allergies: NKDA

• Medications: HCTZ, amitriptyline

• H/O HTN, depression, DM2 ×1 year

FH: None

SH: No ETOH/cig/drug use

Sex H: • Unspecified STD (penile d/c) ×2

• Not currently sexually active

• Erectile dysfunction

Physical Examination

VS: Within normal limits

Gen: Well appearing, NAD

Chest: Clear to auscultation, B/L

CV: Regular rate and rhythm, no murmurs/rubs/gallops, JVP 7 cm

Abd: (+) BS, abd tympanic to percussion all 4 quadrants, no hepatosplenomegaly. No palpable masses; soft, nontender, nondistended. No guarding or rebound tenderness. No CVA or spinal tenderness.

Neuro: • Sensation intact (dull, sharp, proprioception)

• Strength 5/5 sym

• DTRs 2+ sym

• No Babinski present

Ext: No cyanosis, clubbing, edema

Differential Diagnosis

1. Benign prostatic hyperplasia
2. Prostate cancer
3. Chronic prostatitis
4. Medication side effect (amitriptyline → anticholinergic effects; diuretics)
5. Urethral stricture (h/o STD)

(Also, diabetic neuropathy/cytopathy)

Diagnostic Workup

1. Rectal/prostate exam
2. Urinalysis
3. Prostate specific antigen (PSA), BUN, creatinine
4. Cystoscopy/urodynamic studies (including postvoid residual) if above unrevealing
5. Prostate biopsy (if high PSA or suspicious prostate exam)

Practice Case 10

Standardized Patient History-Taking Checklist

1. Where was your weakness? Can you describe it?
2. Which side was your facial droop?
3. Were you confused during, before, or after the episode?
4. Do you feel back to your usual self now?
5. Did you have any slurred speech?
6. Any fevers/chills/chest pain/nausea/seizure activity?
7. Did you now or recently have a loss or change of vision?
8. Have you had any recent falls?
9. Have you had any vertigo, double vision, incontinence?
10. Has this ever happened before?
11. Are you allergic to any medications?
12. Do you take any medications?
13. Do you have any previous illnesses?
14. Does anyone in your family have any major illnesses?
15. Do you smoke, drink, or use illicit drugs?
16. How much do you smoke (for how long)?

Standardized Patient Physical Examination Checklist

1. Examinee washes hands *prior* to examination.
2. Examinee determines patient's mental status and level of alertness.
3. Examinee performs funduscopic examination.
4. Examinee performs cranial nerve examination.
5. Examinee checks motor strength.
6. Examinee checks deep tendon reflexes.
7. Examinee evaluates sensation with at least two modalities (sharp, dull, vibratory).
8. Examinee checks cerebellar function (dysmetria, dysdiadochokinesia, or Romberg).
9. Examinee performs Babinski test.
10. Examinee auscultates lungs.
11. Examinee auscultates precordium in at least two positions.
12. Examinee auscultates carotid arteries.
13. Examinee palpates pulse and/or point of maximal impulse.
14. Examinee auscultates abdomen.
15. Examinee palpates abdomen in all four quadrants.
16. Examinee examines extremities for edema/clubbing/cyanosis.

History

CC   66 yo M c/o weakness, facial droop

HPI: • R facial droop, R arm and R hand weakness, ×20 minutes
          • (+) Dysarthria, (+) confusion
          • (+) Recent amaurosis fugax ×2, R side

- (–) Chest pain, SOB, palpitations
- (–) Fever, chills, falls, vertigo, headaches
- (–) Bowel/bladder incontinence, seizures

PMH:
- One prior episode, 5 min duration, 1 week prior
- Allergies: NKDA
- Medications: lisinopril, ASA, metformin, atorvastatin
- Med h/o HTN, DM, ↑ lipids

FH:
- Noncontributory (adopted)

SH:
- No ETOH/drug use
- (+) 50-pack/year tobacco use

Physical Examination

VS: Hypertensive at 151/90 mm Hg, otherwise within normal limits

Gen: Well appearing, NAD

Ophth/neuro: PERRL, EOM intact, no lesions/papilledema on funduscopic exam

Neuro: A&O ×3, CN II–XII intact, motor 5/5 all muscle groups, DTRs 2+ symmetric, sensation intact to sharp, dull, proprioception. (–) Romberg, (–) dysmetria, (–) Babinski; normal gait.

Chest: Clear to auscultation B/L

CV: Regular rate and rhythm, no murmurs/rubs/gallops, JVP <5 cm. PMI normal size, not displaced. No carotid bruits. Peripheral pulses 2+.

Abd: (+) BS, no palpable masses, soft, nontender, nondistended

Differential Diagnosis

1. Transient ischemic attack
2. Thrombotic or embolic stroke
3. Hypoglycemia or hyperglycemia
4. Seizure disorder
5. Carotid dissection

Diagnostic Workup

1. CT scan of head (brain)
2. Blood glucose
3. Carotid duplex ultrasonography
4. EKG, echocardiogram (if previous studies unrevealing)
5. Electroencephalogram (EEG; if previous studies unrevealing)

Practice Case 11

Standardized Patient History-Taking Checklist

1. Where is the pain located (**Site**)?
2. What is the **Intensity** of the pain?
3. How would you describe the pain (**Quality**)?
4. When did the pain begin (**Onset**)?
5. Does the pain **Radiate**?
6. Is the pain **Associated** with any fevers, movement, weight bearing?
7. Have you had any other joint involvement (**Associated symptoms**)?
8. Have you noticed a rash or other skin changes?
9. Does anything **Alleviate** the symptoms?
10. Does anything **Aggravate** the symptoms?
11. Have you had this before (**Previous episode**)?
12. Do you have any drug **Allergies**?
13. Do you take any **Medications**?
14. Do you smoke, drink, or use illicit drugs (**Social history**)?
15. Does anyone in your family have any major illness or similar symptoms (**Family history**)?
16. Do you have any past medical illnesses, such as hypertension, diabetes, or high cholesterol?
17. What is your diet like (**Social history**)?
18. Are you sexually active (**Sexual history**)?
19. Do you use condoms?

Standardized Patient Physical Examination Checklist

1. Examinee washes hands *prior* to examination.
2. Examinee auscultates lungs.
3. Examinee auscultates precordium in at least two positions.
4. Examinee auscultates abdomen.
5. Examinee percusses abdomen in all four quadrants.
6. Examinee palpates abdomen in all four quadrants.
7. Examinee examines extremities for edema/clubbing/cyanosis/nodules.
8. Examinee feels toe for warmth.
9. Examinee palpates toe for effusion/tenderness.
10. Examinee performs active and passive range of motion exam on toe.
11. Examinee examines other joints for warm/effusion/erosion.
12. Examinee looks at skin for evidence of rash.

History

CC: 40 y/o M c/o L foot pain

HPI: • L foot/great toe pain ×1 day
       • Trauma history (stubbed at night club)
       • 4/10, worse over day → 8/10

- Pain in foot as well, "ache," no other joint involvement
- Pain improved with NSAIDs (indomethacin)
- Worse with walking
- (+) Subjective fever

PMH:
- Two similar events, one requiring ER, given indomethacin
- Allergies: NKDA
- Medications: HCTZ
- Med h/o HTN
- Diet high in shellfish, alcohol, and red meat

FH: Noncontributory

SH:
- No tobacco or drug use
- (+) Moderate ETOH consumption, most days of week, drunk once a week
- (−) CAGE screening
- Pharmaceutical rep

Physical Examination

VS: Low grade fever 100.5 F, hypertensive at 158/90 mm Hg, otherwise WNL

Gen: Well appearing; no apparent distress

Chest: Clear to auscultation, B/L

CV: Regular rate and rhythm, no murmurs/rubs/gallops; (−) JVD

Abd: (+) BS, abd tympanic to percussion all 4 quadrants, no hepatosplenomegaly. No palpable masses; soft, nontender, nondistended.

MS: (+) Pain L great toe with active and passive range of motion, (−) effusion or erythema. No nodules/tophi/bony erosions. No other joint involvement.

Skin: No rash/lesions

Differential Diagnosis

1. Gout
2. Pseudogout (calcium pyrophosphate dihydrate crystal disease)
3. Trauma/Hairline fracture
4. Reactive arthritis
5. Drug side effect (thiazide-induced hyperuricemia and gout)

Diagnostic Workup

1. Joint aspiration
2. Joint fluid crystal analysis/culture/Gram stain/cell count
3. WBC with differential, BUN, creatinine, ESR
4. X-ray of joint
5. Serum uric acid

Practice Case 12

Standardized Patient History-Taking Checklist

1. Where is the pain located? (**Site**)
2. What is the **I**ntensity of the pain? How would you describe it? (**Quality**)
3. When did the symptoms begin? (**Onset**)
4. Does the stomach pain move (**Radiate**)?
5. Have you had any fevers, chills, or diarrhea? (**Associated manifestations**)
6. Have you had any weight loss or gain?
7. Have you had increased urination, hunger, or thirst?
8. Have you had any visual changes?
9. Does anything **A**lleviate or **A**ggravate the symptoms?
10. Has this ever happened before? (**Previous episode**)
11. Are you allergic to any medications? (**Allergies**)
12. Do you take any medications? (**Medicines**)
13. What other medical illnesses and hospitalizations have you had? (**History**)
14. Have you had any dysuria or change in diet? (**Review of systems**)
15. Does anyone in your family have diabetes? (**Family history**)
16. Do you smoke, drink, or use illicit drugs? (**Social history**)
17. Are you sexually active? (**Sexual history**)

Standardized Patient Physical Examination Checklist

1. Examinee washes hands *prior* to examination.
2. Examinee performs funduscopic and ocular exam.
3. Examinee auscultates lungs.
4. Examinee auscultates precordium in at least two positions.
5. Examinee auscultates abdomen.
6. Examinee percusses abdomen in all four quadrants.
7. Examinee palpates abdomen in all four quadrants.
8. Examinee examines extremities for edema/clubbing/cyanosis.
9. Examinee checks sensation in extremities to at least two modalities (sharp, dull or vibratory; diabetic exam).
10. Examinee checks feet for any lesions (diabetic exam).
11. Examinee notes patient discomfort, offers emesis bowl or support or advises to lie down.

History

CC: 26 yo Caucasian M, abd pain, emesis (nonbloody)

HPI:
- Abdominal pain, lethargy ×24 h
- Dull, diffuse, aching pain, 4/10
- (+) Polyuria, polyphagia, polydipsia
- (+) Blurred vision
- (−) Fever, chills, cough, bowel changes, cough, dysuria, sick contacts, diet changes
- No alleviating or aggravating factors
- (+) 10-lb weight loss over few weeks

PMH: • No prior occurrences of similar event

        • Allergies: NKDA

        • Medications: None

        • No other illnesses/hospitalizations

FH: DM two parents and uncle

Sex H: Monogamous with girlfriend, uses condoms

SH: No ETOH/cig/drug use

Physical Examination

VS: RR: 26/min, borderline hypotension with systolic 108 mm Hg; otherwise WNL

Gen: Well appearing; NAD

PERRLA: Normal funduscopic exam

Ophth: PERRL, EOMI, normal funduscopic exam

Neuro: Sensation intact to sharp, dull, vibratory, DTRs 2+, motor 5/5 all muscle groups

Chest: Clear to auscultation B/L, tactile fremitus within normal limits, (+) Kussmaul respi-
        rations (deep, rapid)

CV: Regular rate and rhythm; no murmurs/rubs/gallops

Abd: (+) BS, abd tympanic to percussion all 4 quadrants, no hepatosplenomegaly. No
        palpable masses; soft, nontender, nondistended.

Ext: Normal foot exam, no lesions

Differential Diagnosis

1. New-onset type 1 diabetes mellitus (IDDM)
2. Type 2 diabetes mellitus (NIDDM)
3. Maturity onset diabetes of youth (MODY)
4. Hemochromatosis
5. Glucagonoma

Diagnostic Workup

1. Fingerstick blood glucose
2. Urinalysis (ketonuria, glucosuria), urine microalbuminuria
3. BUN, creatinine, serum glucose, hemoglobin A_{1c}, ketones
4. Ferritin level
5. Somatostatin-receptor scintigraphy (CT or MRI if not available)

KAPLAN
medical

Practice Case 13

Standardized Patient History-Taking Checklist

1. When did this start?
2. How much and how often do you have bowel movements?
3. Is there any pain or discomfort?
4. Can you describe the pain?
5. On a scale of 1/10, how severe is the pain?
6. Any history of dark or bloody stools?
7. Have you had any fevers, chills, or sick contacts?
8. Have you had any rash or skin problems, visual problems, or joint pain?
9. Have you had any weight loss or appetite changes?
10. Have you ever bled before? (**P**revious episode)
11. Are you allergic to any medications? (**A**llergies)
12. Do you take any medications? (**M**edicines)
13. What other medical illnesses and hospitalizations have you had? (**H**istory)
14. Does anyone in your family have any major illnesses, specifically cancer or inflammatory bowel disease? (**F**amily history)
15. Do you smoke, drink, or use illicit drugs? (**S**ocial history)

Standardized Patient Physical Examination Checklist

1. Examinee washes hands *prior* to examination.
2. Examinee examines eyes for evidence of uveitis.
3. Examinee auscultates lungs.
4. Examinee auscultates precordium in at least two positions.
5. Examinee auscultates abdomen.
6. Examinee percusses abdomen in all four quadrants.
7. Examinee palpates abdomen in all four quadrants.
8. Examinee examines skin for any lesions.
9. Examinee examines knees for evidence of inflammation.
10. Examinee examines extremities for edema/clubbing/cyanosis.

History

CC: 35 yo M c/o diarrhea

HPI: • Diarrhea ×1 year
        • Intermittent, occasional gross blood, mucus
        • H/o fecal incontinence
        • 10–20 BM/day
        • Associated with lower abd pain, 4/10, crampy
        • (+) Night sweats, 20-lb weight loss, fever, chills, arthralgias
        • (−) Skin lesions, visual changes, red eyes

PMH:
- No prior occurrences of diarrhea
- H/o perianal fistula
- Allergies: NKDA
- Medications: no Rx, OTC medications, or supplements

FH:
- Uncle ? GI illness → "partial gut resection"
- No known colon cancer

SH:
- No ETOH/cig/drug use
- Married, two healthy children
- Rabbinic student

Physical Examination

VS: Low-grade temp at 100.2, otherwise WNL

Gen: Thin and pale, NAD

Chest: Clear to auscultation, B/L

CV: Regular rate and rhythm, no murmurs/rubs/gallops

Abd: Mild tenderness to palpation RLQ, no guarding or rebound tenderness. Bowel sounds present, tympanic in all four quadrants, no palpable masses or pain on palpation. (−) Murphy sign

Ext: No cyanosis, clubbing, edema; no effusion/inflammation in knees

Differential Diagnosis

1. Crohn disease
2. Ulcerative colitis
3. Colon cancer
4. GI tuberculosis
5. Amebic versus bacterial dysentery

Diagnostic Workup

1. Rectal exam
2. KUB, small bowel series
3. Colonoscopy (or barium enema)
4. Stool for bacterial cultures, ova and parasite exam, occult blood, fecal leukocytes, AFB smear (and place PPD)
5. WBC, AST, ALT, bilirubin, alkaline phosphatase

Practice Case 14

Standardized Patient History-Taking Checklist

1. Where is the pain located? (**S**ite)

2. On a scale of 1 to 10, how intense is the pain? (**I**ntensity/Quantity)

3. Can you describe the pain? (**Q**uality)

4. When did this start? (**O**nset)

5. Any history of dark, bloody, or mucous stools?

6. Have you had any rash or skin problems, visual problems, or joint pain? (**A**ssociated manifestations)

7. Have you had any weight loss, fevers, or appetite changes?

8. Does anything improve your symptoms? (**A**lleviating symptoms)

9. Does anything worsen your symptoms? (**A**ggravating symptoms)

10. Have you had this as a child or teenager? (**P**revious event)

11. Are you allergic to any medications? (**A**llergies)

12. Do you take any medications? (**M**edicines)

13. What other medical illnesses and hospitalizations have you had? (**H**istory of hospitalization/surgery/illness)

14. Does anyone in your family have any major illnesses, specifically cancer or inflammatory bowel disease? (**F**amily history)

15. Do you smoke, drink, or use illicit drugs? (**S**ocial history)

16. Have you had any pregnancies? (**O**b/Gyn)

17. How many children/deliveries?

Standardized Patient Physical Examination Checklist

1. Examinee washes hands *prior* to examination.

2. Examinee examines eyes for evidence of uveitis or thyroid disease.

3. Examinee inspects neck for evidence of goiter.

4. Examinee palpates neck for evidence of goiter.

5. Examinee auscultates lungs.

6. Examinee auscultates precordium in at least two positions.

7. Examinee auscultates abdomen.

8. Examinee percusses abdomen in all four quadrants.

9. Examinee palpates abdomen in all four quadrants.

10. Examinee examines skin for any lesions.

History

CC: 22 y/o F c/o abd pain

HPI:
- Abd pain 5+ years
- Crampy/colicky, diffuse
- 4/10, never wakes patient from sleep
- Associated with diarrhea alternating with constipation
- Stool: + mucus, no blood/melena/acholic stools, normal volume

- (+) Bloating, flatulence
- No weight loss/anorexia/arthralgias/fevers/chills/nausea/GERD/early satiety/visual problems

PMH:
- No prior occurrences of similar event as child/teenager
- Allergies: sulfa, ASA, vitamin C → "headaches"
- Medications: OTC laxatives, antidiarrhea meds
- Past history of depression, treated with SSRI

FH: Unknown, estranged from mother

Ob/Gyn: Twins, vaginal delivery

Sex H: Not sexually active, no h/o STDs

SH: No ETOH/cig
+ Marijuana 1–2×/month

Physical Examination

VS: WNL

Gen: Well appearing, no apparent distress

Ophth: PERRL, EOMI, no stare/lid lag/exophthalmos

Thyroid: (–) Goiter

Chest: Clear to auscultation, B/L

CV: Regular rate and rhythm, no murmurs/rubs/gallops

Abd: (+) BS, abd tympanic to percussion all 4 quadrants, no hepatosplenomegaly. No palpable masses, soft, nondistended. Mildly tender to palpation, without rebound or guarding. Negative Murphy sign.

Skin: No rash/lesions

Differential Diagnosis

1. Irritable bowel syndrome
2. Inflammatory bowel disease (Crohn vs. ulcerative colitis)
3. Pelvic floor dysfunction/rectocele
4. Laxative abuse
5. Hyperthyroidism

Diagnostic Workup

1. Rectal and pelvic exam
2. KUB
3. Flexible sigmoidoscopy
4. WBC, BUN, creatinine, TSH
5. Stool cultures, fecal leukocyte count, examination for ova and parasites, fecal fat

KAPLAN
medical

Practice Case 15

Standardized Patient History-Taking Checklist

1. When did this start?
2. Did these problems start suddenly or gradually?
3. Are things getting better or worse?
4. Have you had any weight loss, anorexia, or night sweats?
5. Do you ever cough up sputum?
6. What does your sputum look like?
7. Have you had any fever, chills, or worsening cough?
8. Do you have chest pain, leg swelling, or shortness of breath when sleeping?
9. What makes your symptoms better?
10. What makes your symptoms worse?
11. Have you ever bled before?
12. Are you allergic to any medications?
13. Do you take any medications?
14. What other medical illnesses and hospitalizations have you had?
15. Does anyone in your family have cancer or any major illnesses?
16. Do you smoke, drink, or use illicit drugs?
17. How long and how much have you smoked?
18. What sort of work did you do?

Standardized Patient Physical Examination Checklist

1. Examinee washes hands *prior* to examination.
2. Examinee performs lymph node exam.
3. Examinee auscultates lungs.
4. Examinee palpates for tactile fremitus.
5. Examinee examines and percusses chest wall.
6. Examinee examines extremities for edema/clubbing/cyanosis.
7. Examinee auscultates precordium in at least two positions.
8. Examinee examines neck for evaluation of jugular venous pressure.
9. Examinee auscultates abdomen.
10. Examinee palpates abdomen in all four quadrants.

History

CC: 65 y/o M c/o breathlessness

HPI: • Progressive dyspnea ×1–2 years
       • Nonproductive cough (scant clear/white sputum), worsening
       • Rare wheeze
       • (+) 30-lb weight loss/6 months, normal appetite
       • No fevers, chills, night sweats, sick contacts
       • No CP, edema, orthopnea
       • Symptoms improve with rest, worse with exertion

PMH: • No prior occurrences of similar event
 • (+) Hypertension
 • Allergies: NKDA
 • Medications: atenolol, ASA

FH: None

SH: • No ETOH, (+) 25 pack-year cigarettes, no drug use
 • Construction worker ×30 years; shipbuilding yard worker in past

Physical Examination

VS: Tachypneic at 24/min, otherwise within normal limits

Gen: Anxious, uncomfortable, thin, pale

Nodes: No cervical/supraclavicular/axillary lymphadenopathy

Chest: Unlabored breathing at 25–30/min, clear to auscultation and percussion B/L, without wheeze, rhonchi, rales, or rubs; (+) cough on expiration/deep inspiration; tactile fremitus within normal limits

CV: Regular rate and rhythm, no murmurs/rubs/gallops, JVP 7 cm

Abd: (+) BS, abd tympanic to percussion all 4 quadrants, no hepatosplenomegaly. No palpable masses, soft, nontender, nondistended.

Ext: (−) Clubbing, cyanosis, edema

Differential Diagnosis

1. Pneumoconiosis (asbestosis vs. silicosis)
2. COPD
3. Lung cancer
4. Mesothelioma
5. Medication side effect (atenolol, aspirin → bronchospasm)

Diagnostic Workup

1. CXR
2. High-resolution CT scan
3. Spirometry with lung volume measurements
4. WBC, arterial blood gas
5. Bronchoscopy with pleural biopsy (dependent on above finding)

Practice Case 16

Standardized Patient History-Taking Checklist

1. Where is the pain located (**Site**)?
2. What is the **I**ntensity of the pain on a scale from 1 to 10?
3. How would you describe the pain (**Quality**)?
4. Are you aware of anything that might have brought this on (**Onset**)?
5. Does the pain move (**Radiate**)?
6. Any nausea or vomiting (**Associated manifestations**)?
7. Any penile discharge, penile lesions, painful or frequent urination?
8. Does anything make the pain better or worse (**Alleviating** and **Aggravating factors**)?
9. Have you ever had this or a similar experience before (**Previous event**)?
10. Do you take any **Medications**?
11. Are you allergic to any medications (**Allergies**)?
12. Are you currently sexually active (**Sexual history**)?
13. Do you use condoms?
14. Is there a history of smoking or drinking (**Social history**)?
15. Do you use any illicit substances?

Standardized Patient Physical Examination Checklist

1. Examinee washes hands *prior* to examination.
2. Examinee asks patient's mother to leave room (tactfully) prior to exam.
3. Examinee auscultates lungs.
4. Examinee auscultates precordium in at least two positions.
5. Examinee auscultates abdomen.
6. Examinee percusses abdomen in all four quadrants.
7. Examinee palpates abdomen in all four quadrants.
8. Examinee examines extremities for edema/clubbing/cyanosis.
9. Examinee palpates knees for effusion/inflammation.
10. Examinee examines skin for lesions/rash.

History

CC: 18 yo M c/o testicular pain

HPI: • Sudden-onset R scrotal pain → groin
        • Pain severe 10/10, woke from sleep
        • (+) Mild abdominal pain, cramping
        • Pain ×4 hours, associated with nausea, nonbloody emesis ×2
        • No fever/chills/penile discharge/lesions/diarrhea/dysuria
        • Mild improvement in pain with elevation/support of testicle
        • Trauma earlier in day, soccer injury
        • Left knee swelling

PMH:
- No prior occurrences of similar event
- Allergies: NKDA
- Medications: None
- No other illnesses

FH: None

Sex H:
- Three female partners, occasional condom use
- (−) STDs/penile discharge/lesions

SH: Rare ETOH (1–2 beers/weekend), no cig/drug use

Physical Examination

VS: Mild tachycardia (105/min)/tachypnea (22/min); otherwise within normal limits

Gen: Moderate discomfort, unable to sit still

Chest: Clear to auscultation B/L

CV: Tachycardic rate and regular rhythm, no murmurs/rubs/gallops

Abd: (+) BS, abd tympanic to percussion all 4 quadrants, no hepatosplenomegaly. No palpable masses; soft, nontender, nondistended.

Ext: No cyanosis, clubbing, edema. No effusion/inflammation either knee

Skin: No rash

Differential Diagnosis

1. Testicular torsion
2. Torsion of appendix testis
3. Orchitis/Epididymitis
4. Trauma (e.g., hematocele, testicular rupture)
5. Henoch-Schönlein purpura (testicular pain, abdominal pain, arthralgias)

Diagnostic Workup

1. Genitourinary exam
2. Urinalysis and urine culture
3. Ultrasound of testicle
4. WBC, BUN, creatinine, ESR
5. Urethral swab (if other studies unrevealing) for *N. gonorrhoeae* and *C. trachomatis*

Practice Case 17

Standardized Patient History-Taking Checklist

1. Where is the pain located (**Site**)?
2. What is the **Intensity** of the pain on a scale from 1 to 10?
3. How would you describe the pain (**Quality**)?
4. Are you aware of anything that might have brought this on (**Onset**)?
5. Does the pain move (**Radiate**)?
5. SOB? Sweating? Nausea or vomiting (**Associated manifestations**)?
6. Does anything make the pain better (**Alleviating factors**)?
7. Does anything make the pain worse (**Aggravating factors**)?
8. Have you ever had this or a similar experience before (**Previous episode**)?
9. Do you have a history of diabetes, hypertension or high cholesterol? Any other medical problems?
10. Do you take any **Medications**?
11. Are you allergic to any medications (**Allergies**)?
12. Are you currently sexually active or have you had any STDs (**Sexual history**)?
13. Is there a history of smoking, drinking, or drug use (**Social history**)? How much?
14. Does anyone in your family have similar problems or related illness/conditions (**Family history**)?

Standardized Patient Physical Examination Checklist

1. Examinee washes hands *prior* to examination.
2. Examinee auscultates lungs.
3. Examinee percusses/palpates chest wall.
4. Examinee feels lungs for tactile fremitus.
5. Examinee auscultates precordium in at least two positions.
6. Examinee examines neck for evaluation of jugular venous pressure.
7. Examinee auscultates carotids for bruits/murmurs.
8. Examinee feels carotid artery pulsation and/or palpates PMI.
9. Examinee checks pulses in extremities.
10. Examinee auscultates abdomen.
11. Examinee palpates abdomen in all four quadrants.
12. Examinee examines extremities for edema/clubbing/cyanosis.

History

CC: 67 yo M c/o CP

HPI:
- CP ×1 hour
- Severe, 10/10, "sharp, tearing"
- Sudden onset while at rest, radiates through to back
- (+) Nausea, diaphoresis, SOB
- (+) Dysphagia, intermittent CP, and nonproductive cough ×1 wk
- (−) Fever, chills, orthopnea, GI, or urinary symptoms
- Not relieved/exacerbated by exertion, little relief with OTC aspirin, acetaminophen

PMH:
- Pain somewhat similar to previous MI
- H/o CAD s/p MI 2 years prior, HTN, STDs, hyperlipidemia; denies DM
- Allergies: NKDA
- Medications: aspirin, atenolol, atorvastatin, HCTZ

FH: None, specifically no early heart disease

SH:
- No ETOH/drug use
- Approx. 75 pack-year h/o tobacco use

Sex H: Not currently sexually active, h/o syphilis and gonorrhea

Physical Examination

VS: Febrile, hypertensive, tachycardic, tachypneic: T 100.8 F, BP 195/115 mm Hg, HR 110/min, RR 30/min

Gen: Anxious, moderate discomfort

Chest: Clear to auscultation and percussion B/L, no reproducible pain, tactile fremitus within normal limits

CV: Tachycardic rate and regular rhythm, no murmurs/rubs/gallops, JVP 8 cm; pulses 2+ B/L, no carotid bruits. PMI not displaced. Normal carotid upstroke and amplitude.

Abd: (+) BS, abd tympanic to percussion all 4 quadrants, no hepatosplenomegaly. No palpable masses, soft, nontender, nondistended

Ext: 2+ pedal pulses, bilaterally. No cyanosis. Motor and sensory function intact.

Differential Diagnosis

1. Dissecting aortic aneurysm (consider luetic thoracic aneurysm)
2. Acute MI
3. Unstable angina
4. Esophageal disruption
5. Pulmonary embolus

Diagnostic Workup

1. CPK, CPK-MB, troponin
2. TEE (transesophageal echocardiography)
3. CXR
4. EKG
5. WBC, hematocrit, arterial blood gas

Practice Case 18

Standardized Patient History-Taking Checklist

1. When did this start?
2. Can you describe the sensation of dizziness?
3. Do you have any associated symptoms?
4. Specifically, how are your hearing, vision, and balance?
5. When do these spells occur, and how long do they last?
6. Are these symptoms worse with movement/positional changes?
7. Have you ever had these symptoms before?
8. Are you allergic to any medications?
9. Do you take any medications?
10. What other medical illnesses and hospitalizations have you had?
11. Have you ever had a seizure?
12. Have you had any weight, appetitive, or gastrointestinal changes?
13. Does anyone in your family have cancer or any major illnesses?
14. Do you smoke, drink, or use illicit drugs?

Standardized Patient Physical Examination Checklist

1. Examinee washes hands *prior* to examination.
2. Examinee checks head for trauma/external lesions.
3. Examinee performs otoscopic exam.
4. Examinee performs Weber test.
5. Examinee performs Rinne test.
6. Examinee performs penlight eye exam.
7. Examinee checks for nystagmus.
8. Examinee visualizes oropharynx.
9. Examinee palpates neck for goiter/lymphadenopathy.
10. Examinee checks cranial nerves.
11. Examinee tests sensation to light touch and pinprick.
12. Examinee tests muscle strength.
13. Examinee evaluates cerebellar reflexes (either finger/nose, gait, Romberg, or dysdiado-chokinesis)
14. Examinee checks deep tendon reflexes.
15. Examinee auscultates carotids.
16. Examinee auscultates precordium in at least two locations.

History

CC: 43 yo F c/o dizziness

HPI: • Vertigo, gradual onset ×6 months
        • Tinnitus, hearing loss
        • Episodes last 20 minutes to few hours
        • "Fullness" L ear

- Worse with position changes
- No fever, chills, trauma, headaches, seizure-like activity, nausea, wt/appetite changes

PMH:
- No prior occurrences of similar event
- Past h/o depression, HTN
- Allergies: NKDA
- Medications: aspirin, atenolol

FH: None

SH: No ETOH/cig/drug use

Physical Examination

VS: Bradycardic at 50/min, otherwise within normal limits

HEENT: Normocephalic, atraumatic; *eyes:* EOMI, PERRL, physiologic nystagmus; *ears:* normal canals and tympanic membrane, (–) pain with movement of pinna; *nose:* normal turbinates; oropharynx: no erythema/exudates/lesions/vesicles; *neck:* supple, no lymphadenopathy or goiter

Neuro: A&O ×3, good concentration. Cranial nerves II–XII intact. (+) Weber, lateralizes to R side; (+) Rinne, air greater than bone conduction, R > L. Motor 5/5 symmetric. Sensation intact to sharp and dull. DTRs 2+ symmetric. Normal Romberg, normal gait, no dysmetria.

CV: No carotid bruits; normal S1, S2 with no murmurs, rubs, or gallops

Differential Diagnosis

1. Ménière disease
2. Benign paroxysmal positional vertigo
3. CNS lesion or mass
4. Atypical seizures
5. Posterior circulation stenosis

Diagnostic Workup

1. Audiometry
2. Vestibular testing
3. Caloric stimulation
4. CT scan or MRI
5. Serum sodium, chloride, bicarbonate, BUN, creatinine, ASA level

Practice Case 19

Standardized Patient History-Taking Checklist

1. When did this start?
2. Where is the pain located?
3. What is the intensity of the pain on a scale from 1 to 10?
4. How would you describe the pain?
5. Have you had any weight loss?
6. Does anything make your symptoms better?
7. Does anything make your symptoms worse?
8. Have you ever had this or a similar experience before?
9. Do you take any medications?
10. Have you suffered anorexia or weight loss?
11. Have you noticed any changes in your urine or bowel movements?
12. Are you currently or in the past sexually active?
13. Do you (did you) use condoms or ever have an STD?
14. Is there a history of smoking or drinking?
15. Have you used intranasal cocaine or injection drugs?
16. Does anyone in your family have similar problems or related illness/conditions?

Standardized Patient Physical Examination Checklist

1. Examinee washes hands *prior* to examination.
2. Examinee auscultates lungs.
3. Examinee looks at chest for evidence of gynecomastia.
4. Examinee auscultates precordium in at least 2 positions.
5. Examinee auscultates abdomen.
6. Examinee percusses abdomen in all four quadrants.
7. Examinee specifically measures liver span and checks for splenomegaly.
8. Examinee palpates abdomen in all four quadrants.
9. Examinee checks for presence of Murphy sign.
10. Examinee looks at skin for signs/stigmata of liver disease.
11. Examinee examines extremities for edema/clubbing/cyanosis.

History

CC: 47 y/o M c/o nausea, fatigue

HPI:
- Gradual onset nausea, fatigue, RUQ pain ×1 year
- Pain 4/10, dull, constant, no radiation
- Tea-colored urine ×1 wk
- Arthralgias, knees and elbows ×1 wk
- (+) 20-lb weight loss ×2 months, anorexia
- (−) Rash, visual changes, fevers, chills, GI, or urinary changes

PMH:
- No prior occurrences of similar event, previously healthy, h/o alcoholism × 5–10 years
- Allergies: NKDA
- Medications: acetaminophen

FH: Uncle: liver failure?

SH:
- Homeless, lives in shelter, unemployed
- Heavy alcohol use, last drink today after weeklong binge
- Past h/o IVDU (heroin)

SexH:
- Not currently sexually active
- Past h/o STDs, multiple sexual partners without condoms

Physical Examination

VS: Within normal limits

Gen: Malnourished, appears older than stated age, (+) jaundice

Chest: Clear to auscultations B/L, no gynecomastia

CV: Regular rate and rhythm, no murmurs/rubs/gallops

Abd: (+) BS, tympanic to percussion all 4 quadrants, no hepatosplenomegaly. RUQ tenderness, but no guarding, rebound, or Murphy sign. No shifting dullness, fluid wave, or bulging flanks.

Skin: No lesions, spider angiomata, or other stigmata of liver disease; two prison tattoos

Ext: No cyanosis, clubbing, palmar erythema, or edema

Differential Diagnosis

1. Alcoholic hepatitis versus chronic viral hepatitis (risk factors for B and C)
2. Acetaminophen toxicity
3. Acute versus chronic pancreatitis
4. Hepatocellular carcinoma
5. Hemochromatosis (family history)

Diagnostic Workup

1. WBC, hematocrit, BUN, creatinine, calcium, ALT, AST, bilirubin, alkaline phosphatase, GGT, PT/INR, PTT
2. HCV antibody, HBsAg, HBsAb, HBcAb
3. Amylase, lipase (if elevated, also add calcium, LDH, glucose), acetaminophen level
4. RUQ ultrasound
5. Alpha-fetoprotein, ferritin level

Practice Case 20

Standardized Patient History-Taking Checklist

1. Can you describe your loss of consciousness? (Did you black out versus feel weak?)
2. Did you feel strange prior to this or notice a precipitating event?
3. Did you feel strange after this event?
4. Any chest pain, shortness of breath, or palpitations?
5. Did you loose control of bladder or bowel function, bite your tongue, or convulse?
6. Did you feel nauseous or sweaty after the event?
7. When you fell, did you hit your head?
8. Was this event witnessed by anyone else?
9. Has anything like this happened before?
10. Are you allergic to any medications?
11. Do you take any medications?
12. What other medical illnesses and hospitalizations have you had?
13. Does anyone in your family have any major illnesses, specifically heart disease?
14. Do you smoke, drink, or use illicit drugs?
15. How much do you smoke?

Standardized Patient Physical Examination Checklist

1. Examinee washes hands *prior* to examination.
2. Examinee palpates/examines skull for trauma.
3. Examinee auscultates lungs.
4. Examinee auscultates precordium in at least two positions.
5. Examinee auscultates carotid arteries for bruits.
6. Examinee examines neck for evaluation of jugular venous pressure.
7. Examinee auscultates abdomen.
8. Examinee percusses abdomen in all four quadrants.
9. Examinee palpates abdomen in all four quadrants.
10. Examinee examines extremities for edema/clubbing/cyanosis.
11. Examinee evaluates gait or Romberg sign.
12. Examinee checks for presence/absence of Babinski sign.
13. Examinee evaluates muscle strength and DTRs.

History

CC: 66 yo F c/o LOC

HPI: • Syncopal episode
        • Occurred while working, upon standing
        • 30-second duration, preceded by nausea, followed by confusion
        • (−) Head trauma, CP, SOB
        • (+) Palpitations earlier in AM
        • (−) Bowel/bladder incontinence, tongue biting, prolonged confusion

PMH:
- HTN, DM, CAD S/P MI, 5 years ago
- No prior occurrences of similar event
- Allergies: NKDA
- Medications: ASA, atenolol, metformin, lisinopril

FH: Heart disease (early MI), DM2

SH:
- No ETOH
- No drug use
- Approximately 25-pack-year history tobacco use

Physical Examination

VS: Bradycardic at 50/min, otherwise WNL

Gen: Well appearing, no apparent distress

Chest: Clear to auscultation, B/L

CV: Bradycardic rate and regular rhythm, no murmurs/rubs/gallops, no JVD, no carotid bruits, PMI not displaced

Abd: (+) BS, abd tympanic to percussion all 4 quadrants, no hepatosplenomegaly. No palpable masses, soft, nontender, nondistended.

Neuro: A&O ×3, good concentration, attentiveness. Motor 5/5 sym., sensation intact to pinprick and light touch, DTRs 2+ sym. (−) Babinski, Romberg, normal gait.

Differential Diagnosis

1. Vasovagal syncope
2. Orthostatic hypotension (diabetic autonomic neuropathy versus beta-blocker)
3. Cardiac syncope due to arrhythmia
4. "Silent" MI
5. Neurogenic syncope/seizures

Diagnostic Workup

1. CPK, CPK-MB, troponin, glucose, HbA_{1c}, hematocrit
2. EKG
3. Event recorder/Holter monitor
4. Tilt table test (if diagnosis unclear)
5. Orthostatics

Practice Case 21

Standardized Patient History-Taking Checklist

1. When did this start?
2. Did these problems start suddenly or gradually?
3. Are things getting better or worse?
4. Have you had any weight loss, anorexia, or night sweats?
5. Do you ever cough up sputum?
6. What does your sputum look like?
7. Have you had any fevers?
8. Do you have chest pain or tightness, palpitations, shortness of breath, or leg swelling?
9. What makes your symptoms better?
10. What makes your symptoms worse?
11. Are you allergic to any medications?
12. Do you take any medications?
13. Are you taking your medications as prescribed?
14. What other medical illnesses and hospitalizations have you had?
15. Does anyone in your family have cancer or any major illnesses?
16. Do you smoke, drink, or use illicit drugs?
17. How long and how much have you smoked?
18. What sort of work did you do?

Standardized Patient Physical Examination Checklist

1. Examinee washes hands *prior* to examination.
2. Examinee performs lymph node exam.
3. Examinee auscultates lungs.
4. Examinee palpates for tactile fremitus.
5. Examinee examines and percusses chest wall.
6. Examinee examines extremities for edema/clubbing/cyanosis.
7. Examinee auscultates precordium in at least two positions.
8. Examinee examines neck for evaluation of jugular venous pressure.
9. Examinee auscultates abdomen.
10. Examinee palpates abdomen in all four quadrants.

History

CC: 66 yo M c/o cough and fever

HPI: • Worsening cough, fever ×3 days
       • H/o chronic productive cough, but now with foul-smelling, greenish sputum
       • (+) Hemoptysis (trace amount), intermittent chest tightness, wheeze
       • (+) Fatigue, 10–20-lb weight loss over 2–3 months
       • (–) Chills, night sweats, chest pain, palpitations, nausea

PMH: •   Past h/o PNA ×2 (hospitalized), pulmonary embolus, COPD, HTN

      •   Allergies: NKDA

      •   Medications: atenolol, warfarin, ipratropium

FH: None

SH: •   No ETOH/drug use

      •   40-pack-year tobacco use

Physical Examination

VS: Febrile at 101 F, hypertensive at 146/90 mm Hg, tachycardic at 107/min, tachypneic at 28/min

Gen: Anxious, uncomfortable, thin, pale, leaning forward

Nodes: No cervical/supraclavicular/axillary lymphadenopathy

Chest: RR of 25–30/min, no accessory muscle use, clear to auscultation and percussion B/L, without wheeze, rhonchi, rales, or rubs. (+) Cough on expiration/deep inspiration; tactile fremitus WNL

CV: Tachycardic rate and regular rhythm, S1/S2, no murmurs/rubs/gallops, JVP 7 cm

Abd: (+) BS, abd tympanic to percussion all four quadrants, no hepatosplenomegaly. No palpable masses, soft, nontender, nondistended

Ext: No cyanosis, clubbing, or edema

Differential Diagnosis

1. Acute exacerbation of chronic bronchitis
2. Community-acquired pneumonia
3. Pulmonary embolus
4. CHF
5. Lung cancer

Diagnostic Workup

1. CXR
2. ABG and pulse oximetry
3. Sputum cultures and sputum cytology
4. WBC, hematocrit, serum sodium, chloride, bicarbonate, BUN, creatinine; consider blood cultures, D-dimer
5. CT angiography or ventilation/perfusion scan

Practice Case 22

Standardized Patient History-Taking Checklist

1. Where is the pain located?
2. What is the intensity of the pain?
3. How would you describe the pain?
4. When did the pain begin? Is it getting worse?
5. Does the stomach pain spread to any other part of your body?
6. Is the pain related to eating?
7. Is the pain associated with nausea, changes in stool color or consistency, fever, or other symptoms?
8. Have you had weight loss, loss of appetite, change in skin or eye color, or fatigue?
9. Does anything alleviate the symptoms?
10. Does anything aggravate the symptoms?
11. Have you had this before?
12. Do you take any medications, specifically NSAIDs or antacids?
13. Do you smoke, drink, or use illicit drugs? How much?
14. Does anyone in your family have any major illness or similar symptoms?

Standardized Patient Physical Examination Checklist

1. Examinee washes hands *prior* to examination.
2. Examinee checks eyes for scleral icterus.
3. Examinee checks for abnormal lymph node (specifically left supraclavicular).
4. Examinee auscultates lungs.
5. Examinee auscultates precordium in at least two positions.
6. Examinee examines neck for presence of JVD.
7. Examinee auscultates abdomen.
8. Examinee percusses abdomen in all four quadrants.
9. Examinee palpates abdomen in all four quadrants.
10. Examinee checks for presence of Murphy sign or palpable gallbladder.
11. Examinee examines extremities for edema/clubbing/cyanosis.
12. Examinee inspects skin for lesions/rash.

History

CC: 51 yo M c/o abdominal pain

HPI:
- 3-month h/o dull, constant epigastric pain
- 4–5/10, radiates to back
- Insidious onset, progressive
- Improvement (mild) with leaning forward, worse with recumbency or eating
- (+) Early satiety, 15-lb weight loss ×1 month, fatigue, anorexia
- (−) Fever, nausea, reflux, CP, change in bowel habits, urinary symptoms

PMH:
- No previous episodes of current symptoms
- Allergies: NKDA
- Medications: None
- Past h/o acute pancreatitis (? etiology), thrombophlebitis, borderline hyperglycemia

FH:
- No family h/o cardiac or gastric disease

SH:
- + 30–60 pack-year tobacco use
- No drug use, rare social ETOH use (1–3 beers/weekend)

Physical Examination

VS: Within normal limits

Gen: No apparent distress, nonjaundiced

HEENT: Scleral icterus

Nodes: No cervical, supraclavicular, or axillary lymphadenopathy

Chest: Clear to auscultation B/L, tactile fremitus normal

CV: S1/S2 normal, no murmurs, rubs, or gallops; no JVD

Abd: Mild tenderness to palpation epigastrium, no guarding or rebound tenderness. Bowel sounds present, tympanic in all four quadrants, no palpable masses or pain on palpation. Neg. Murphy sign. Nonpalpable gallbladder.

Skin: No lesions

Ext: No peripheral edema, cyanosis, clubbing

Differential Diagnosis

1. Pancreatic cancer
2. Biliary carcinoma
3. Duodenal carcinoma
4. Chronic pancreatitis
5. Peptic ulcer disease

Diagnostic Workup

1. Rectal exam with stool exam for occult blood
2. Spiral CT scan or MRI of abdomen
3. WBC, hematocrit, amylase, lipase, liver function tests
4. Upper endoscopy (if not available, upper GI barium series)
5. ERCP or MRCP
6. CEA level, CA 19-9 level (depending on previous studies)

Practice Case 23

Standardized Patient History-Taking Checklist

1. Is there any associated pain?
2. How often do you see blood in your urine?
3. Is the blood most prominent at the beginning, middle, end, or throughout urination?
4. Are you aware of anything that might have brought this on?
5. Do you suffer from weight loss, diminished appetite, fatigue, or pain?
6. Do you suffer from flank pain, fevers, chills, urinary urgency or frequency?
7. Does anything improve your symptoms?
8. Does anything make the pain worse?
9. Have you ever had this or a similar experience before?
10. Do you take any medications or have any medication allergies?
11. Do you have a past medical history of UTIs or kidney stones?
12. Have your eating habits changed in any way?
13. Does anyone in your family have similar problems or related illness/conditions?
14. Are you currently sexually active? Any history of sexually transmitted diseases?
15. Is there a history of smoking or drinking?
16. Do you exercise regularly or vigorously?

Standardized Patient Physical Examination Checklist

1. Examinee washes hands *prior* to examination.
2. Examinee auscultates lungs.
3. Examinee auscultates precordium in at least two positions.
4. Examinee auscultates abdomen.
5. Examinee percusses abdomen in all four quadrants.
6. Examinee palpates abdomen in all four quadrants.
7. Examinee checks for costovertebral angle tenderness, flank masses.
8. Examinee examines extremities for edema/clubbing/cyanosis.

History

CC: 60 yo M hematuria

HPI: • 3 episodes gross hematuria over 3 mo
        • Painless, lasts entire episode of micturition
        • No clear precipitating events
        • No clear alleviating/aggravating factors
        • 3 mo h/o dysuria, frequency, nocturia, urgency
        • (−) Pain, anorexia, fever, chills, weight loss, flank pain

PMH: • No prior occurrences of similar event
        • Allergies: NKDA
        • Medications: ASA
        • Prior h/o renal calculi ×1, 5 years prior. No dietary changes

FH: • None, no known malignancies

• Sex H: No STDs, monogamous with wife ×35 years

SH: • No ETOH/cig/drug use

• Runs 5–10 miles, 4 days/week

• No occupational exposures

Physical Examination

VS: Within normal limits

Gen: Well appearing, NAD

Chest: Clear to auscultation, B/L

CV: Regular rate and rhythm, no murmurs/rubs/gallops

Abd: (+) BS, abd tympanic to percussion all four quadrants. No palpable masses, soft, nontender, nondistended. No surgical scars

Back: No CVA tenderness, masses

Ext: No clubbing, cyanosis, edema

Differential Diagnosis

1. Bladder (or other uroepithelial) cancer
2. Benign prostatic hyperplasia
3. Glomerulonephropathies
4. Urinary tract infection
5. Renal/bladder calculi

Diagnostic Workup

1. Genitourinary and rectal exam
2. Urine for cytology, urinalysis, and culture
3. Cystoscopy
4. Intravenous pyelogram
5. CT scan of abdomen and pelvis

Practice Case 24

Standardized Patient History-Taking Checklist

1. When did this start?
2. Did the symptoms start suddenly or gradually?
3. How would you describe the weakness and fatigue? Are they located in any particular place?
4. Are your symptoms constant or intermittent?
5. Does anything make your symptoms better?
6. Does anything make your symptoms worse?
7. Have you noticed any associated symptoms?
8. Specifically, have you had visual changes, focal weakness, pain, arthralgias, or heat/cold intolerance?
9. Have you ever had this or a similar experience before?
10. Do you have any medical problems?
11. Do you take any medications?
12. Have you noticed any changes in urination?
13. Have your eating habits changed in any way? Changes in bowel habits?
14. Does anyone in your family have similar problems or related illness/conditions?
15. Are you currently sexually active?
16. Is there a history of smoking, drinking, or drug use?

Standardized Patient Physical Examination Checklist

1. Examinee washes hands *prior* to examination.
2. Examinee inspects and correctly palpates thyroid gland (patient asked to swallow).
3. Examinee performs lymph node exam.
4. Examinee auscultates lungs.
5. Examinee auscultates precordium in at least two positions.
6. Examinee auscultates abdomen.
7. Examinee percusses abdomen in all four quadrants.
8. Examinee palpates abdomen in all four quadrants.
9. Examinee examines extremities for edema/clubbing/cyanosis.
10. Examinee performs cranial nerve exam with focus on EOM and papillary response.
11. Examinee evaluates motor strength.
12. Examinee evaluates sensation with sharp and dull stimuli.
13. Examinee evaluates deep tendon reflexes.
14. Examinee checks for Babinski sign.

History

CC: 24 yo F c/o weakness

HPI: • Weakness and fatigue ×2 months
        • Gradual onset, no clear precipitating event, constant weakness and fatigue
        • (+) Blurry vision/diplopia, (+) intermittent jaw/tongue weakness
        • Difficulty chewing and swallowing

- Symptoms worse with using stairs, eating, exertion
- No alleviating factors known
- (–) Rash, fever, chills, arthralgias, recent illnesses, seizures
- (–) Heat/cold intolerance, diarrhea, constipation, palpitations
- (–) Weight changes, polyphagia, polyuria, depressed mood

PMH:
- No prior occurrences of similar event
- Allergies: NKDA
- Medications: OCP
- No past medical history

FH:
- Mother: thyroid condition ? ("neck gland problem")

SH:
- No ETOH/cig/drug use
- Grad student, mechanical engineering

Physical Examination

VS: WNL

Gen: Well appearing, NAD

Ophth: EOMI, PERRL, conjugate gaze, no inducible ptosis

Neck: No thyromegaly by inspection or palpation

Nodes: No cervical, supraclavicular, or axillary lymphadenopathy

Chest: Clear to auscultation, B/L

CV: Normal S1, S2. Regular rate and rhythm; no murmurs/rubs/gallops

Abd: (+) BS, abd tympanic to percussion all four quadrants, no hepatosplenomegaly. No palpable masses; soft, nontender, nondistended

Neuro: A&O ×3, compliant with exam. CN II–XII intact. Motor: 5/5 in all muscle groups. Sensation intact to light touch/pinprick. DTRs 2+ symmetrically

Differential Diagnosis

1. Myasthenia gravis
2. Lambert-Eaton syndrome
3. Botulism
4. Hypo/hyperthyroidism
5. New onset diabetes (blurred vision, weakness)

Diagnostic Workup

1. Tensilon (edrophonium) test
2. Acetylcholine receptor antibody titers, Lambert-Eaton autoantibody titers (presynaptic Ca channel antibodies)
3. Blood glucose, TSH
4. Nerve conduction studies
5. EMG

Practice Case 25

Standardized Patient History-Taking Checklist

1. When did this start?
2. Was the onset sudden or gradual?
3. Do you have trouble getting or maintaining an erection?
4. Do you still have a desire for sex?
5. Do you have trouble with premature or painful ejaculation?
6. Does this problem occur all the time or just occasionally?
7. Do you masturbate or have nocturnal/morning erections?
8. Have you noticed any associated symptoms?
9. Specifically, any painful urination, pain or discharge (nipple or penile), visual changes, or breast enlargement?
10. How are you and your spouse getting along?
11. How are your mood, energy, stress, anxiety, and enjoyment levels?
12. Does anything make your symptoms better?
13. Does anything make your symptoms worse?
14. Have you ever had this or a similar experience before?
15. Do you have a history of diabetes, alcoholism, hypertension, drug abuse, or other medical problems?
16. Do you take any medications?
17. Have you ever had a sexually transmitted disease?
18. Is there a history of smoking or drinking?
19. How much do you drink or smoke (drinks/day, packs/day)?
20. Does anyone in your family have similar problems or related illness/conditions?

Standardized Patient Physical Examination Checklist

1. Examinee washes hands *prior* to examination.
2. Examinee performs confrontational visual field exam.
3. Examinee inspects and correctly palpates thyroid gland.
4. Examinee auscultates lungs.
5. Examinee palpates/inspects chest wall for breast changes/discharge.
6. Examinee auscultates precordium in at least two positions.
7. Examinee auscultates for bruits.
8. Examinee palpates peripheral pulses.
9. Examinee auscultates abdomen.
10. Examinee percusses abdomen in all four quadrants.
11. Examinee palpates abdomen in all four quadrants.
12. Examinee examines extremities for edema/clubbing/cyanosis.
13. Examinee checks for diabetic complications (either neuropathy, retinopathy, and/or diabetic foot exam).
14. Examinees performs checks for motor and sensory function in extremities.

History

CC: 68 yo M c/o inability to have sex with wife (erectile dysfunction)

HPI: • Difficulty getting and maintaining erection, failure/pain with ejaculation ×8 months
        • Gradual, progressive, constant onset
        • Reduced libido, denies masturbation, questionable nocturnal/AM erections
        • (+) Fatigue, constipation
        • (+) Anxiety over health, heart condition
        • (−) Dysuria, testicular/penile pain, discharge, gynecomastia, nipple discharge, heat/cold intolerance, visual changes, or poor relationship with spouse
        • (−) Depressed mood, sleep disturbances, anhedonia
        • No alleviating or aggravating factors

PMH: • No prior occurrences of similar event
        • Allergies: NKDA
        • Medications: ASA, metoprolol, metformin, lisinopril
        • Past h/o DM2, HTN, CAD, s/p MI 1 year ago

FH: • Father died of MI in 60s, mother with DM

SxH: • No STDs, monogamous with wife ×40 years

SH: • (+) ETOH: 1–2 drinks/day ("highball"), (+) 50+ pack-year tobacco use, (−) drugs

Physical Examination

VS: WNL

Gen: Well appearing, NAD

Ophth: No visual field defects, formal fundus

Endo: No goiter by inspection or palpation

Chest: Clear to auscultation B/L, no gynecomastia/nipple discharge

CV: Regular rate and rhythm, no murmurs/rubs/gallops, pulses 2+, no carotid or abdominal bruits

Abd: (+) BS, abd tympanic to percussion all four quadrants, no hepatosplenomegaly. No palpable masses; soft, nontender, nondistended

Ext: Good muscle bulk, intact sensation to pinprick/light touch. No cyanosis/clubbing/edema, no lesions/ulcerations

Differential Diagnosis

1. Vascular disease (diabetic versus CAD complication)
2. Psychogenic (fear of cardiac event, anxiety over son, depression)
3. Androgen deficiency (hypothalamic versus pituitary versus testicular)
4. Drug-induced erectile dysfunction
5. Hypothyroidism

Diagnostic Workup

1. GU and prostate exam
2. Hemoglobin A_{1c}/fasting glucose level (assess diabetic control)
3. TSH, testosterone, prolactin levels
4. Nocturnal penile tumescence testing ("postage stamp test")
5. Duplex penile ultrasonography, followed by penile angiography (depending on above results)

Practice Case 26

Standardized Patient History-Taking Checklist

1. Where is the pain located?
2. What is the intensity of the pain on a scale from 1–10?
3. How would you describe the pain? Sharp or dull?
4. Are you aware of anything that might have brought this on?
5. Does the pain spread anywhere?
6. How would you describe your visual loss (monocular vs. scotoma)?
7. How would you describe your jaw pain?
8. Does your jaw pain get worse or better with continued use?
9. Any warning signs, triggers, or aura?
10. Does anything make the pain better?
11. Does anything make the pain worse?
12. Have you ever had this or a similar experience before?
13. Are you under stress or suffer from depression or anxiety?
14. Do you take any medications?
15. Is there a history of smoking or drinking?
16. Does anyone in your family have similar problems or related illness/conditions?

Standardized Patient Physical Examination Checklist

1. Examinee washes hands *prior* to examination.
2. Examinee inspects and palpates temporal region of scalp.
3. Examinee checks papillary response and extraocular muscles.
4. Examinee performs funduscopic exam.
5. Examinee performs otoscopic exam and palpates pinnae.
6. Examinee palpates neck for lymphadenopathy.
7. Examinee auscultates lungs.
8. Examinee auscultates precordium in at least two positions.
9. Examinee auscultates abdomen.
10. Examinee palpates abdomen in all four quadrants.
11. Examinee examines extremities for edema/clubbing/cyanosis.
12. Examinee evaluates cerebellar function (gait, finger/nose, or Romberg).
13. Examinee checks cranial nerves.
14. Examinee checks muscle strength and cutaneous sensation.
15. Examinee assesses deep tendon reflexes.
16. Examinee assesses for presence of Babinski sign.

History

CC: 62 yo F c/o HA, jaw pain, visual problems

HPI:
- Intermittent L HAs ×6 months
- 6/10 intensity, sharp or dull/throbbing, quick onset
- Daily attacks, can last ×1 hr
- Radiates to front of head and nape of neck
- No clear triggers, slightly worse with movement/position/exercise
- Mild improvement with ASA
- (+) Amaurosis fugax, jaw claudication
- (+) Fevers, 15-lb weight loss, fatigue/malaise
- (−) Joint pain, nausea, aura, focal weakness, photophobia, halos

PMH:
- No prior occurrences of similar event
- Allergies: NKDA
- Medications: ASA, metoprolol, NTG
- Past h/o CAD, angina, HTN

FH:
- Mother with migraines

SH:
- No ETOH/cig/drug use
- Works as corporate lawyer, high stress level, good mood

Physical Examination

VS: Low-grade fever at 100.8 F, hypertensive at 158/70 mm Hg, otherwise within normal limits

Gen: Ill-appearing, pale, but comfortable

HEENT: Normocephalic, atraumatic, (+) L temporal tenderness without palpable cord; (−) TMJ/auricular tenderness. EOMI, PERRL, (−) funduscopic abnormalities or papilledema, (−) otoscopic abnormalities with normal canals and clear tympanic membranes. Neck supple, no lymphadenopathy

Chest: Clear to auscultation, B/L

CV: Regular rate and rhythm, no murmurs/rubs/gallops, no carotid or temporal bruits

Abd: (+) BS, abd tympanic to percussion all four quadrants, no hepatosplenomegaly. No palpable masses, soft, nontender, nondistended

Ext: Full range of motion, no cyanosis, clubbing, edema

Neuro: A&O ×3, good concentration. CN II-XII intact. Strength 5/5 all muscle groups, DTRs 2+. Sensation intact to sharp and dull stimuli. Normal gait (tandem), finger/nose, (−) Romberg.

Differential Diagnosis

1. Temporal arteritis
2. TMJ disorder vs. dental disease
3. Medication rebound headache vs. side effect (beta-blockers, nitroglycerin)
4. Muscle tension
5. Migraine headache

Diagnostic Workup

1. ESR, C-reactive protein
2. Snellen vision test
3. WBC, complete blood count
4. X-ray of TMJ
5. Temporal artery biopsy

Practice Case 27

Standardized Patient History-Taking Checklist

1. When did this start?
2. Was the onset sudden or gradual?
3. Is the discharge copious and constant or intermittent?
4. How would you describe the consistency of the discharge?
5. How would you describe the odor of the discharge?
6. What color is the discharge?
7. Is there any blood?
8. Is there any pain, itchiness, fever, weight loss, or pelvic pain?
9. Are you aware of anything that might have brought this on?
10. Does anything make your symptoms better or worse?
11. Have you ever had this or a similar experience before?
12. Do you have a history of diabetes or other medical problems?
13. Do you take any medications?
14. Are you currently sexually active?
15. Do you have a history or STDs? Do you use condoms?
16. Have you had a Pap smear?
17. Is there a history of smoking or drinking?
18. Does anyone in your family have similar problems or related illness/conditions?

Standardized Patient Physical Examination Checklist

1. Examinee washes hands *prior* to examination.
2. Examinee auscultates lungs.
3. Examinee auscultates precordium in at least two positions.
4. Examinee auscultates abdomen.
5. Examinee palpates abdomen in all four quadrants.
6. Examinee inspects skin for any rash or other lesion.

History

CC: 30 yo F c/o vaginal discharge

HPI:
- 1-wk thick, frothy discharge, intermittent
- Green, white, occasionally yellow discharge, questionable trace blood
- No clear precipitating event (note: recent new tampon use)
- (+) Odor: "fishy," pruritic, pelvic "fullness"? subjective low-grade fevers
- (−) Weight change, pelvic pain, fatigue, rash
- No alleviating/aggravating factors

PMH:
- No prior occurrences of similar event
- IDDM, h/o DKA 2 years ago
- Allergies: None
- Medications: NPH/regular insulin SQ BID

FH:
- None. Parents and sister alive and well

OB/GYN:
- No children/pregnancies, LMP 2 weeks ago, normal. Can't remember last GYN visit; never had Pap smear

SexH:
- Uses condoms "sometimes," no STDs, sexually active with boyfriend

SH:
- No cig/drug use, rare ETOH

Physical Examination

VS: WNL

Gen: Well appearing, NAD

Chest: Clear to auscultation, B/L

CV: Regular rate and rhythm, no murmurs/rubs/gallops

Abd: (+) BS, abd tympanic to percussion all four quadrants, no palpable masses, soft, non-tender, nondistended

Skin: No rash

Differential Diagnosis

1. *Trichomonas*
2. Vulvovaginal candidiasis
3. Bacterial vaginosis
4. Acute cervicitis (gonorrhea vs. chlamydia)
5. Retained foreign body (tampon, condom)

Diagnostic Workup

1. Bimanual and speculum exam
2. KOH and saline prep
3. WBC, β-hCG
4. Swab and smear for culture and sensitivity, *Trichomonas*, *Gardnerella*
5. Pap smear

Practice Case 28

Standardized Patient History-Taking Checklist

1. When did this start?
2. Have your symptoms been constant or intermittent?
3. Are you aware of anything that might have brought this on?
4. Have you had difficulty concentrating?
5. Do you hear voices or see things that others can't?
6. Have you had difficulty at work or with friends and family?
7. Do you feel hot, flushed, or have changes in skin/hair/bowel habits?
8. Does anything seem to make things better or worse?
9. Have you ever had this or a similar experience before?
10. Do you take any medications?
11. Do you have any past medical problems?
12. Have you had any psychiatric or mood problems?
13. Is there a history of smoking or drinking?
14. Do you use any illicit substances or herbal supplements?
15. Does anyone in your family have similar problems or related illness/conditions?

Standardized Patient Physical/Mental Status Examination Checklist

1. Examinee washes hands *prior* to examination.
2. Examinee evaluates alertness and orientation.
3. Examinee evaluates speech pattern.
4. Examinee tests recent and distant memory.
5. Examinee asks patient to repeat serial sevens to test concentration/attention.
6. Examinee evaluates patient's mood and affect.
7. Examinee asks about perception—hallucinations, delusions, and paranoias.
8. Examinee specifically asks if patient wants to hurt self or others.
9. Examinee asks if patient understands the condition and its implications (judgment/insight).
10. Examinee inspects and palpates thyroid.
11. Examinee auscultates lungs.
12. Examinee auscultates precordium in at least two positions.
13. Examinee auscultates abdomen.
14. Examinee percusses and palpates abdomen in all four quadrants.

History

CC: 22 yo F c/o difficulty sleeping

HPI:
- 2 weeks decreased need for sleep, heart racing
- (+) Racing thoughts, increased energy and goal-directed behavior
- (+) Grandiosity at work, shopping sprees, excessive verbosity
- (−) Fevers, heat/cold intolerance, hair loss, skin changes, bowel/bladder changes
- (−) Hearing voices, visions

PMH: • No prior occurrences of similar event

     • Past h/o depression, episodic palpitations/diaphoresis

     • Allergies: None

     • Medications: None

FH: • No medical/psychiatric history

SH: • Denies cig/drug use

     • (+) ETOH, unclear quantity

     • ? Promiscuity (multiple new boyfriends)

Physical Examination

VS: WNL

Gen: A&O ×3, well groomed, obviously agitated and can't sit still

Psych: Speech pressured, but fluid and goal directed. Recent and remote memory is intact. Attention and concentration normal by serial sevens. Euphoric mood, consistent affect. Normal perceptions without hallucination, delusions, paranoias. Denies suicidal/homicidal ideations. Poor insight and judgment

Neck: No goiter by inspection/palpation

Chest: Clear to auscultation B/L

CV: Regular rate and rhythm, no murmurs/rubs/gallops

Abd: (+) BS, abd tympanic to percussion all four quadrants, no hepatosplenomegaly. No palpable masses; soft, nontender, nondistended

Skin: No lesions/changes

Differential Diagnosis

1. Bipolar disorder/mania
2. Schizophrenia
3. Hyperthyroidism
4. Amphetamine abuse
5. Alcohol withdrawal

Diagnostic Workup

1. TSH and free T_4
2. Urine toxicology screen
3. Blood alcohol level

Practice Case 29

Standardized Patient History-Taking Checklist

1. When did this start?
2. Was the onset sudden or gradual?
3. Has the diarrhea been constant or intermittent?
4. How much diarrhea has there been?
5. Does the stool contain blood or mucus? Foul-smelling?
6. Are you aware of anyone else with these symptoms?
7. Does the child attend daycare?
8. Has anything improved or worsened the symptoms?
9. Has there been any nausea?
10. Does your child appear to be in pain?
11. Have you noticed any changes in behavior or other symptoms?
12. Does the child take any medications?
13. Has the child been able to tolerate fluids/foods?
14. Has there been any change in your child's diet?
15. Have there been any previous episodes of diarrhea?
16. Has your child traveled anywhere?
17. Does anyone in your family have similar problems or related illness/conditions?

History

CC: Mother 1 y/o M child, not available for physical exam

HPI: • 3 day h/o watery diarrhea
        • Constant, large volume (fill diaper)
        • Associated with nonbloody, greenish vomit
        • ? Episode of blood/mucus
        • Low-grade temperature, irritable
        • Daycare sick contacts
        • Recent trip to India
        • Birth/prenatal history: vaginal delivery at 39 weeks, full prenatal care
        • Growth/development: normal growth/development, age-appropriate milestones met
        • Immunizations: age-appropriate immunizations

PMH: • No prior occurrences of similar event
        • Allergies: none
        • Medications: pediatric acetaminophen, oral rehydration solution
        • No dietary changes prior to event, difficulty tolerating PO intake

FH: • No ill family members, no smokers in household

Differential Diagnosis

1. Rotavirus vs. Norwalk vs. other virus
2. Bacterial gastroenteritis (*Shigella, Salmonella, Escherichia coli*)
3. Parasitic gastroenteritis (*Giardia, Amoeba, Cryptosporidia*)
4. Food poisoning (*Staphylococcus, Clostridium*)
5. Intussusception

Diagnostic Workup

1. Physical examination of child
2. Rectal examination (stool exam for blood/mucus)
3. WBC with differential, hematocrit
4. Stool for microscopic exam, culture, toxin
5. KUB, barium enema

Practice Case 30

Standardized Patient History-Taking Checklist

1. When did this start?
2. When does the discharge occur?
3. Is the discharge in one or both breasts?
4. Is it thick or thin?
5. What color is the discharge?
6. Is blood present?
7. Is an odor present?
8. Does anything make the symptoms better or worse?
9. Have you had any pain, fevers, chills, heat/cold intolerance, or other symptoms?
10. Have you checked for a breast lump?
11. Have you had any symptoms (discharge, pain, mass) in the other breast?
12. Have you ever had this or a similar experience before?
13. Do you have any illnesses?
14. Do you take any medications (birth control pills)?
15. Does anyone in your family have similar problems, related conditions, or cancer?
16. Are you currently sexually active?
17. When was your last menstrual period?
18. Is there a history of smoking, drinking, or drug use?

Standardized Patient Physical Examination Checklist

1. Examinee washes hands *prior* to examination.
2. Examinee inspects and correctly palpates thyroid gland.
3. Examinee palpates lymph nodes (cervical, supraclavicular, and axillary).
4. Examinee auscultates lungs.
5. Examinee auscultates precordium in at least two positions.
6. Examinee auscultates abdomen.
7. Examinee percusses and palpates abdomen in all four quadrants.
8. Examinee examines extremities for edema/clubbing/cyanosis.

History

CC: 32 yo F c/o nipple discharge

HPI: • Nipple discharge ×2 wks, L breast
        • Occurs intermittently most mornings
        • Thin consistency, odorless, small amount ("drops")
        • Green tint, occasionally milky, one episode of blood
        • Denies pain, heat/cold intolerance, fevers, trauma, symptoms in contralateral breast
        • No new lump noted, h/o "lumpy breasts," questionable increase in size

PMH: • No prior occurrences of similar event
        • Allergies: NKDA
        • Medications: none

FH: • Mom—ovarian cancer, deceased age 40s
        • Dad—DM, alive
        • Aunt—breast cancer, deceased age 40s

GYN :   • LMP 2 weeks ago, normal; sexually active with boyfriend, (+) condoms

SH: • No ETOH/cig/drug use

Physical Examination

VS: WNL

Gen: Well appearing, NAD

Thyroid: No goiter

Nodes: No cervical, supraclavicular, or axillary lymphadenopathy

Chest: Clear to auscultation B/L

CV: Regular rate and rhythm, no murmurs/rubs/gallops

Abd: (+) BS, abd tympanic to percussion all four quadrants, no hepatosplenomegaly. No palpable masses; soft, nontender, nondistended

Skin: Normal, no lesions

Differential Diagnosis

1. Breast carcinoma (intraductal vs. lobular)

2. Duct ectasia versus papilloma

3. Prolactinoma

4. Pregnancy (physiologic discharge, though usually bilateral)

5. Hyperthyroidism

Diagnostic Workup

1. Breast examination

2. Diagnostic mammogram, breast ultrasound, and chest radiograph

3. Fluid cytology

4. Fine needle biopsy (if mass present on exam)

5. Free T_4 and TSH level, serum prolactin, pregnancy test, genetic (BRCA) testing

Practice Case 31

Standardized Patient History-Taking Checklist

1. When did this start?

2. Are your symptoms constant most of the day?

3. Are things getting better or worse?

4. Do you still enjoy your hobbies and interests (anhedonia)?

5. Do you suffer from fatigue or loss of energy?

6. Do you feel worthless or guilty?

7. Do you have difficulty concentrating?

8. Do you think of death or suicide?

9. Does anything make these thoughts better or worse?

10. Have you ever had this or a similar experience before?

11. Do you take any medications?

12. Do you have a history of medical or psychiatric illnesses?

13. Have you had any change in your sleep pattern?

14. Have your eating habits changed in any way?

15. Are there any illnesses or psychiatric symptoms that run in your family?

16. Is there a history of smoking, drinking, or drug use?

17. How much do you drink?

Standardized Patient Physical/Mental Status Examination Checklist

1. Examinee washes hands *prior* to examination.
2. Examinee evaluates alertness and orientation.
3. Examinee evaluates speech pattern.
4. Examinee tests recent and distant memory.
5. Examinee asks patient to repeat serial sevens to test concentration/attention.
6. Examinee evaluates patient's mood and affect.
7. Examinee asks about perception—hallucinations, delusions, and paranoias.
8. Examinee specifically asks if patient wants to hurt self or others.
9. Examinee asks if patient has *plan* to hurt self/others.
10. Examinee asks if patient is aware of his condition and its implications (judgment/insight).
11. Examinee inspects and palpates thyroid.
12. Examinee auscultates lungs.
13. Examinee auscultates precordium in at least two positions.
14. Examinee auscultates abdomen.
15. Examinee percusses and palpates abdomen in all four quadrants.

History

CC: 54 y/o M c/o crying all the time

HPI: • 1 year depressed mood, decreased energy
        • Crying spells daily
        • (+) Anhedonia, anorexia, alienation from friends/family, insomnia
        • (+) Weight loss (15 lbs/6 months), sense of worthlessness
        • (–) Heat/cold intolerance, constipation, skin/hair changes
        • (–) Precipitating event
        • (–) Alleviating/aggravating factors

PMH: • No prior occurrences of similar event
        • Allergies: NKDA
        • Medications: aspirin, atenolol, prednisone
        • Past h/o CAD s/p MI ×1 year, HTN, rheumatoid arthritis

FH: • No psychiatric history, (+) heart disease, DM
        • SH: No tobacco use, h/o drug use (? current drug use)
        • (+) ETOH "2–3 highballs" per day

Physical Examination

VS: WNL

Gen: Well appearing, NAD

Psych: Appearance–well groomed, A&O ×3. Speech–mildly slow and goal directed. Recent and remote memory is intact. Attention and concentration reduced, tested by serial sevens. Depressed mood, consistent affect. Normal perceptions without hallucination, delusions, paranoias. Denies homicidal ideations. (+) suicidal ideations, no plan or time frame. Good insight and judgment

Neck: Thyroid normal to inspection and palpation

Chest: Clear to auscultation, B/L

CV: Regular rate and rhythm, no murmurs/rubs/gallops

Abd: (+) BS, abd tympanic to percussion all four quadrants, no hepatosplenomegaly. No palpable masses; soft, nontender, nondistended

Differential Diagnosis

1. Unipolar major depression
2. Drug/alcohol use
3. Medication side effect (beta-blocker, corticosteroids)
4. Hypothyroidism vs. subclinical hypothyroidism
5. Diabetes mellitus

Diagnostic Workup

1. Drug screen
2. Blood alcohol level
3. Free T_4 and TSH level
4. Fasting blood glucose

Practice Case 32

Standardized Patient History-Taking Checklist

1. When did this start?
2. Was the onset sudden or gradual?
3. How severe are your symptoms—are you able to eat a meal?
4. Where does the food appear to get stuck?
5. When does the food get stuck (beginning or end of swallow)?
6. Is it more difficult to swallow solids or liquids?
7. Is there any pain associated with swallowing?
8. Have you suffered from fevers, nausea/vomiting, weight loss, or fatigue?
9. Have you had any dark stools, foul breath, or hoarse voice?
10. Does anything make your symptoms better or worse?
11. Have you ever had this or a similar experience before?
12. Are you allergic to any medications?
13. Do you take any medications?
14. Do you have any medical illnesses?
15. Does anyone in your family have similar problems or related illness/conditions?
16. Is there a history of smoking or drinking?
17. How much did you smoke and drink?

Standardized Patient Physical Examination Checklist

1. Examinee washes hands *prior* to examination.
2. Examinee inspects oropharynx and orocavity.
3. Examinee correctly inspects and palpates thyroid.
4. Examinee palpates cervical and supraclavicular lymph nodes.
5. Examinee auscultates lungs.
6. Examinee auscultates precordium in at least two positions.
7. Examinee examines neck for evaluation of jugular venous pressure.
8. Examinee auscultates abdomen.
9. Examinee percusses abdomen in all four quadrants.
10. Examinee palpates abdomen in all four quadrants.
11. Examinee examines extremities for edema/clubbing/cyanosis.

History

CC: 52 yo M c/o difficulty swallowing

HPI: • 1 month h/o progressive dysphagia
        • Solids but not liquids, severe
        • Location deep in throat, present after swallowing initiated
        • Intermittent pain not directly associated with swallowing
        • Pain retrosternal, 4/10, "burning"
        • (+) Halitosis, 15-lb weight loss/1 month, fatigue, melena, hoarseness